Healthy Joints for Life

Healthy Joints for Life

An Orthopedic Surgeon's Proven Plan
to Reduce Pain and Inflammation,
Avoid Surgery and Get Moving Again

RICHARD DIANA, M.D.
WITH SHEILA CURRY OAKES

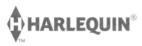

Healthy Joints for Life

ISBN-13:978-0-373-89270-9

© 2013 by Richard Diana

Illustrations by John M. Havel

Line drawings by Janet Croog

The health advice presented in this book is intended only as an informative resource guide to help you make informed decisions; it is not meant to replace the advice of a physician or to serve as a guide to self-treatment. Always seek competent medical help for any health condition or if there is any question about the appropriateness of a procedure or health recommendation.

Library of Congress Cataloging-in-Publication Data

Diana, Richard, 1960–
Healthy joints for life: an orthopedic surgeon's proven plan to reduce pain and inflammation, avoid surgery and get moving again/Richard Diana, M.D.; with Sheila Curry Oakes.

 pages cm
Includes bibliographical references.
ISBN 978-0-373-89270-9
1. Joints—Diseases—Popular works. 2. Pain—Popular works. 3. Arthritis—Popular works. I. Title.
RC932.D528 2013
616.7'2—dc23
          2013008832

www.Harlequin.com

Printed in U.S.A.

For my mom and dad

For my precious Ann, Jack, and Megan

For all my patients, who continue to inspire and educate me

And for all of us who seemingly came from nothing
Who scratched and fought for what we have
And, at some point, realized we came from everything

CONTENTS

APPENDIX II

INTRODUCTION

LET ME TELL YOU ABOUT MY MOTHER. BY THE TIME I GRADUATED from medical school, my sixty-two-year-old mother had already suffered through several surgeries for her rheumatoid arthritis (RA), a despicable form of arthritis where the body attacks its own joints as it would invading bacteria. The resulting inflammatory response is incredibly intense. Multiple joints swell, hurt, and degenerate.

Her treatments were torturous. Regular injections of gold and methotrexate gave her nausea and headaches but didn't reduce her pain. Anti-inflammatory medicines gave her an ulcer. Nothing stopped the aggressive progression of her joint pain and joint destruction.

I was a budding doctor, working around the clock to learn all the answers about how to treat and heal medical conditions. Seeing her suffer from the disease was excruciating. Seeing the treatments make her worse was beyond heart-wrenching. I desperately wanted to help, but her aggressive RA wasn't going to wait for me or medical research. Or anything else. After treatments with countless medications failed miserably, she had surgery to reroute and repair ruptured hand tendons. Her left wrist had to be fused. As a result, she fed herself with difficulty and could barely hold a cup of water. Even before the hand surgeries, standing had become so painful that the ends of several eroded bones in both of her feet had to be removed. Like a relentless tide, the disease slowly but persistently ate away at her joints.

By her seventieth birthday her knees were bone on bone and her hips were equally bad. Her inactivity led to other medical problems, like diabetes and heart disease, so she wasn't healthy enough to have replacement surgery, and she could barely walk by the end. Sadly, my most intimate moments with my mom consisted of me draining the fluid from her swollen knees and shoulders. RA deprived my mother of some of the best days of her life, and all I could do was watch in horror. I was a grown man, a surgeon, and an ex–NFL player, and I cried for my mother—and my kids saw me. They saw my mother, they saw my helplessness, and they understood what RA was doing to all of us.

Because of my mother, I came to hate inflammation and joint pain and what they can do to a person. I will never forget what they did to my mother.

***

For four decades I've been witnessing the devastating effects of inflammation and joint pain both personally and professionally. For years I've been studying the science behind inflammation and devising ways to defeat it. I now have a battle-tested, scientifically sound game plan to deal with joint pain and inflammation.

As for this book, it will be my job to make the science behind joint pain understandable and interesting. I will spare you most of the gory details but will arm you with enough knowledge so you can better understand what is happening to your joints and how my program will help them. I'll tell you some stories from the NFL, college football, and my medical training and practice. I'll keep it simple and clear. Once you understand my program and put the plan into action, you will start to get your life back. You will start controlling your joint pain, and your joint pain will stop controlling you.

MOM AND DAD, THE SUPER BOWL, AND LEADERSHIP

Almost every day of my life as an orthopedic surgeon, I'm asked what it was like to play in the Super Bowl. It always amazes me how important and alluring that one event is. Many of my patients think it's cool that I'm the only orthopedic surgeon to have ever played in the Super Bowl, but the Super Bowl has much greater importance to me than that.

The play-offs for the 1982 season were the first time that my parents ever flew on a plane. Those few weeks were some of the most exciting weeks of their lives. They were on TV, were interviewed by reporters, and were treated like royalty all because their son was playing for the Miami Dolphins in Super Bowl XVII. They came to practices, took pictures with legendary Dolphin coach Don Shula, and met the guys on the team. They sat on the fifty-yard line. For a short time they were treated like the celebrities that I always thought they were, and that meant more to me than anything.

The thing I remember most about the Super Bowl was a conversation that I had right before the game with the captain of our team, Bob Kuechenberg, or "Kooch," as we knew him. Kooch was making the rounds, trying to make sure everybody was ready. He approached me and said, "Rookie, you've been doing it all year for us. Now it's time to help the other guys do it, too." It was just five seconds of encouragement accompanied by a tap on the back. But it made me think like I hadn't before about my role as a player and a leader. It was time for me to step forward and become a team leader. The Super Bowl was the day when I realized that *following* was not enough. Though football was the earlier and greater passion in my life, medicine became my ultimate vocation. Helping people would be my life's mission. Going through medical school, internship, and residency took a long ten years, and as a med student, intern, and resident, I was closely monitored and rigorously tested along the way. In school I wasn't exactly in a position to be a leader. But over the past two decades, I've helped a lot of people, and with this book I hope to help many more. Of course, Kooch couldn't have known what direction my life would take, but I'm convinced that when he spoke to me right before the Super Bowl, his words foreshadowed that my ultimate accomplishment would be leading people with joint pain toward pain relief.

In 2010 the Miami Dolphins invited players from the 1983 and 1985 Super Bowl teams for a reunion. Since my retirement twenty-seven years prior to the reunion, I'd been back to Miami only once, for Dan Marino's retirement celebration. On the flight down I thought of all the sweat, pain, and violence we, as players, endured during our quest for the Super Bowl. We learned that success in football comes from dedication, intensity, focus, and passion. It was understood that while we might lose, we would never be outworked. We had an incredible commitment to one another and, of course, to winning. I shuddered as I thought about what we did to our bodies to play the game of football—to win.

It was wonderful to reunite with my teammates. In so many ways nothing had changed, and in so many other ways everything had changed. After retiring from the NFL I became an orthopedic surgeon, applying many of the principles learned from football to helping those with musculoskeletal problems. At the reunion, I learned quickly that most of my teammates suffered terribly from years of abusing their bodies. Several had knee and hip replacements, two had back fusions, most suffered with neck arthritis, and virtually everyone limped or at least complained of joint pain. Some had put on a few—or more!—pounds. Previous studies on ex–NFL players revealed that those extra pounds were often associated with life-threatening heart disease. I worried about these men, who, decades ago, were my family.

All of us had aged in those intervening decades, and in talking with my teammates, I realized that I had the ability to do something to help them not only with their joint pain but also with a potential scare: heart disease. Those talks with my teammates spawned the idea for this book.

During many nights of research and writing, it became obvious that while my teammates inspired *Healthy Joints for Life,* this book is long overdue for anyone and everyone who has joint pain and wants to avoid surgery. As an added bonus, the diet, exercise, and supplement recommendations are heart-healthy and reduce cancer, too.

I am confident that *Healthy Joints for Life* will reduce your joint pain and improve the quality of your life and perhaps even its length! With each chapter, the reward of joint-pain relief and improved health is that much closer. When you can walk on a beach or visit a museum without pain, you will be thankful. When you can make the long walk from the parking lot to see your children or grandchildren play a sport, you will know it's worth it.

Now that you know a little bit about my background, let's take advantage of my discoveries and get to work making your joints feel better.

PART ONE

Understanding
Joint Pain

CHAPTER 1

INFLAMMATION:
The Cornerstone of Disease

I'M GOING TO START YOU ON THE ROAD TO JOINT-PAIN RELIEF with one simple statement: to control joint pain, you need to control inflammation. Get used to hearing about inflammation, because you are going to learn more about it than you ever imagined. Before you finish this book, you will understand many molecular details of inflammation, as well as some of the most obvious outward symptoms of joint pain, and how and why inflammation drives it. You are going to learn that when you reduce inflammation, you will significantly reduce your joint pain.

Inflammation is part of the body's mechanism of fighting infection, responding to irritants or injuries, and initiating healing. It comes in many forms. Its manifestations can be as straightforward as the swelling of a sprained ankle or as subtle as the slow, insidious development of joint-surface wear and tear that we call arthritis. Sometimes inflammation is good and necessary. In fact, inflammation plays a key role in the life-sustaining process of fighting infections. But in the case of joint pain, inflammation becomes excessive and it doesn't know when to stop. It's out of control, kind of like I was when I played on special teams for the Miami Dolphins.

BUSTING THE WEDGE

Despite being small by NFL standards, I played on a lot of special teams for the Dolphins. One of my tasks was being a wedge buster on kickoffs. The wedge buster is the guy who runs down the field as hard as he can—talk about overzealous—and slams into the opponent's "wedge" of big, tough behemoths who block for the kickoff returner. After smashing the wedge, he tries to tackle the ballcarrier.

The job of wedge buster is usually reserved for the craziest guys on the football team. Typically, these guys are beasts who are not on a life path to Mensa. Their marbles are a bit shaken up, partially because their brains were scrambled by gigantic hits while playing on special teams and partially because, well, they started out a little crazy. To run down the field at absolute full speed and slam into an opponent without regard to the well-being of your own body or your opponents' takes a certain perversity—not to mention a total disregard for life and limb. (Unfortunately, we are learning through research that by sustaining gigantic hits while playing on special teams, there may be future devastating brain effects.)

Well, there I was, a Yale graduate and a molecular biophysics and biochemistry major, and I had all sorts of regard for life and limb, but at the same time, I had a job to do. Oddly enough, I loved that job. I loved the contact, the intensity, and the camaraderie. Much more so than the average guy, I loved to smash into people.

During the last preseason game of 1982 I was sent out to wedge bust against the New York Giants. I was the second man to the right of the kicker, a prime spot for making tackles. Before each kickoff I tried to work myself into a frenzy by reciting some of Clint Eastwood's lines from *The Outlaw Josey Wales*. "When things look bad, and it looks like you're not gonna make it, then you gotta get mean. I mean plumb mad-dog mean. 'Cause if you lose your head and you give up, then you neither live nor win. That's just the way it is." Other guys would psych themselves up by whacking their helmets until their ears rang. I psyched myself up by reciting lines from Clint Eastwood movies. I never looked at my routine as particularly crazy, but I guess in some ways I was really different from many of my teammates.

So there I was, reciting Clint Eastwood lines, smashing into freakishly large and strong brutes, fearing for my life, loving every minute of it, and at the other end of the kickoff was the Giants' mega-money first-round draft pick—a big, fast running back out of the University of Michigan named Butch Woolfolk.

Woolfolk caught the ball at the goal line, at least ten yards to my left, and within five strides he was running full out. A hole opened at the fifteen-yard line, and Butch was nearly through it when I closed on him from the opposite side and hit him full speed with my helmet, like a battering ram.

Butch went flying five yards sideways with three twists and a flip. Fireworks went off in my head. Proudly, I staggered off the field with a serious headache. With a touch of Clint Eastwood, a lot of effort, and a hard head I helped stop the Giants and Butch Woolfolk.

Now it's time for you to use your head in a completely different manner to stop inflammation and joint pain. With a touch of knowledge, a lot of discipline, and the help of diet, exercise, and supplements, you are going to control inflammation and pain.

CONTROLLING INFLAMMATION

The way we control inflammation is by controlling the way cells use molecules to communicate inflammatory signals.

This probably sounds complicated and technical, but don't worry. I'm not going to take you through all the biochemistry behind cells and molecules and how they work to create inflammation. I'm simply going to help you understand what inflammation does to the body—particularly your joints—and how it can be reduced and potentially stopped.

THE SCIENCE OF INFLAMMATION

Nearly any injury or disease that strikes the body involves inflammation. Inflammation afflicts the heart with heart disease and other organs with cancer. It can be the reason why your teeth fall out or why your toe hurts when you stub it.

What's ironic is that although there are multiple diseases where inflammation plays a role, inflammation is still a mystery to many. Mainstream doctors haven't fully embraced the inflammatory theory of disease or spread the news to the public, because when most doctors went through medical school, they weren't taught about the impact of inflammation on the body. That is starting to change and will continue to change over the next decade, particularly because, more and more, inflammation is being identified as the core cause of so many diseases and illnesses. In 2013 the Blavatnik Family Foundation awarded $10 million to Yale immunobiologists to investigate the role of inflammation as a "theory of everything" for disease! Philanthropist Leonard Blavatnik believes this concept "represents a paradigm shift in the science of chronic disease...."

Remember, inflammation isn't all bad. We could not cope or survive without the inflammatory cycle. If we stopped inflammation completely, we would die. That's why my program seeks to balance inflammation. Swelling is an important part of the inflammatory process. The right amount of swelling facilitates healing. Too much swelling slows healing. Trauma is a typical cause of swelling, but trauma isn't the only cause of swelling or inflammation. Sometimes inflammation sneaks up on us, because it begins at the cellular level and we don't feel it until it causes a joint to swell, degenerate, and hurt;

heart arteries to narrow and clog (heart attack); lung airways to constrict (asthma); or damaged cells to multiply out of control (cancer).

What causes inflammation? Mechanical stresses from obesity, pollution, job stress, fast foods, and food additives, to name a few. Over time, these irritants can deviously brew in our cells, leading to many insidious diseases, including joint arthritis. A key to maintaining health is balancing the positive and negative effects of inflammation. And the most significant negative effect of inflammation that I want to eliminate, or at least reduce, is joint pain.

Our overall health and the reduction of joint pain are dependent upon keeping inflammation in balance. Monitoring inflammation is a 24-7 job. By following my program, you'll balance inflammation and reduce joint pain.

CELLS

Cells are the individual building blocks of our organs. Organs communicate and interact with one another so that the body functions as a whole. For example, the lungs and heart communicate and interact with every breath and beat. Specifically, lungs deliver oxygen to the blood so the heart can pump oxygenated blood throughout the body. They work together as a unit. One of the many fascinating functions of the body is the intricate interaction that occurs among bones, muscles, cartilage, ligaments, and the joint lining—all of which have cells that communicate and interact, just like organs do.

Cells in our bones, muscles, ligaments, and cartilage have to talk to each other in order to work. But cells don't always get the message straight. Unfortunately, for some of us, those erroneous, overaggressive messages lead to joint pain.

Osteoarthritis used to be considered solely a disease of joint cartilage, that rubbery tissue that covers and cushions the end of bones. It is now known to be a disease of all the elements of the joint: the synovial lining, bone, cartilage, muscle and ligaments, not to mention the immune system's white blood cells. This way of thinking is referred to as the whole joint theory of osteoarthritis. Treating osteoarthritis, and therefore treating joint pain, means addressing the inflammatory balance of all the cells of the entire joint, not just the cartilage. Understanding this concept has led to significant changes in how I attempt to treat the disease. The target of treatment is no longer only cartilage. Treatment has expanded to include all the elements of the joint. Each essential element of the joint must be efficiently and effectively treated. Nutrition, exercise/movement, and supplements can be manipulated to reach down into the cells of the joints that are so intimately involved in causing joint pain. Joint pain from osteoarthritis isn't solely mechanical. Arthritis is more than wear and tear. The debilitating pain of arthritis starts at the cellular level, and that is why it is so important for us to thoroughly understand cell structure, the mechanisms of cell inflammation, and how cells communicate.

Cells communicate with each other with incredible precision. However, sometimes cells make mistakes, and it's up to us to correct them. The mistakes are not intentional—just biological. When a cell needs to communicate, it sends out swift wireless molecular messages, and it does so ingeniously, miraculously, and clearly. If a joint infection occurs, for example, joint cells quickly contact the immune system by producing chemical messages in the form of protein molecules, which are released through the outer wrapping of the cell, called the cell membrane.

Cell Membranes

A cell membrane is like a police line. It lets the good stuff in and out but keeps the bad stuff at bay on both sides of the barricade. It must be versatile enough to maintain a lightning-fast, orderly, and constant flow of molecules in and out of the cell. A cell membrane is made primarily of fat (lipids) and cholesterol. It's an odd combination, especially when you consider that the fats and cholesterol in the membrane are stacked in layers, like a double-layered birthday cake. Fat serves as the building blocks for establishing a supple, flowing, dynamic compartment to contain the cell contents. Cholesterol adds some rigidity to the compartment. A mixture of saturated fats and unsaturated fats keeps the cell membrane functioning at optimum levels. Too much cholesterol and the cell membrane is too rigid; too much saturated fat and the cell membrane is too firmly packed. With the right amount of cholesterol, saturated fat, and unsaturated fat, you will have a fluid, communicative cell membrane.

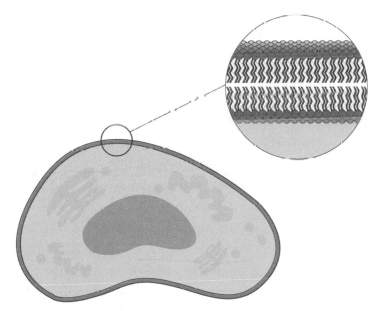

Membrane science is not so simple, however. The fats making up the membrane are the building blocks for the messengers of inflammation and anti-inflammation. Saturated and omega-6 unsaturated fats in the membrane can be processed into inflammatory messengers, and omega-3 unsaturated fats can be processed into anti-inflammatory messengers. Therefore, fat, that same stuff that plagues our midsections, needs to be understood all the way down to the molecular level, because some fats can be part of the joint pain solution, while others represent a part of the problem. The fats that make up the cell membrane, referred to as phospholipids, deserve our attention.

The system of cell communication works ingeniously. In order for the cell membrane to allow the right "stuff" in and out of the cell, its security system has to be precise. Necessary chemical messengers enter and exit with a quick flash of a molecular key or ID card. Once in the cell these chemical messengers can stimulate cell processes, such as the inflammatory process we so desperately want to control.

Eating healthy proteins, sugars, and fats is very important to maximize cell performance. Because cell membrane makeup can be influenced by what we eat, it is important that we consume the right foods. In Chapter 3, you will learn much more about the foods that can significantly reduce inflammation. For now, suffice it to say that what you eat has a direct impact on how well your cells function and, in turn, how well your body functions.

If you follow health news or pay attention to food ads, you have probably heard about the fats known as omega-3s or omega-6s. Eating predominately omega-6 fatty acids (found in a variety of foods including refined vegetable oils and margarine) will cause your cell membranes to be overly populated with these fatty acids that trigger inflammation. Omega-3 fatty acids (primarily found in fish and nuts) are the starting blocks for anti-inflammatory chemical messengers, which balance the effects of the inflammatory messengers. Basically, it's up to the omega-3s to fight off the inflammatory nature of the omega-6s.

If you consume a specific joint-healthy diet featuring more omega-3 fatty acids and less omega-6 fatty acids cell membranes will be more favorably balanced. This simple dietary manipulation will help your joints. In Chapter 3 we will add upon this concept to further advance our mission of joint-pain relief. Learn the concepts, and your joints will thank you for it.

THE INFLAMMATORY PATHWAYS

There is a chain of events that can transform the fats in cell membranes into agents of inflammation. Prescription medications (Mobic, Celebrex) and over-the-counter medications (Advil, Aleve, and aspirin) chemically modify the pathways that form inflammatory messengers—but so do omega-3 fatty acids, which we can find in food. Mobic, Celebrex, Advil, Aleve, and aspirin can all suppress inflammatory messengers, but aspirin can also transform specific inflammatory messengers into protective messengers, aptly called protectins and resolvins. So if you absolutely have to reach for the pill bottle, aspirin seems to offer an advantage over the other anti-inflammatories. This program is going to help minimize such a need, but I realize that at some point we all seek pain relief through medication. Remember that, despite being easily obtained, all over-the-counter medications (Advil, Aleve, and aspirin) can cause ulcers and internal bleeding, so we need to be very careful how often we use them. My program will teach you to go to the kitchen, instead of the medicine cabinet, for long-term relief from joint pain and inflammation.

A QUICK MENTION OF ASPIRIN ✓

Research on aspirin and heart disease has directed many middle aged men to include an 81 mg aspirin in their daily health regimen. Certainly this is not appropriate for every man because aspirin can have significant side effects. Contraindications include blood thinners, a history of ulcers, gastrointestinal problems, or certain neurological conditions. The beneficial consequence for all those taking aspirin for heart health is that it is also beneficial for joint health. Those who suffer from joint pain get the

continued

benefit that aspirin has on a specific inflammatory enzyme called the COX-2 enzyme (see Chapter 2 and "The Inflammatory Pathways" section in Appendix I). Aspirin modifies the COX-2 enzyme, which leads to the production of resolvins and protectins from omega-3s. Resolvins resolve inflammation, and protectins protect from inflammation. (See Appendix I for more details.) For men without contraindications, the benefits may outweigh the risks, making a baby aspirin a day a no-brainer. Results for women (Ridker 2005) are somewhat less compelling, probably due to the hormones that are different in men and women. Talk to your cardiologist about this. Helping your heart may also help your joints!

In addition to the omegas, there are other fats that can either positively or negatively impact inflammation on the cellular level. In future chapters we'll talk about saturated and unsaturated fats in detail. The worst fatty acid for your cell membranes is trans-fatty acid, which can be found in vegetable shortenings and in some margarines, crackers, cookies, fried foods, and snack foods. New York has banned them. These detrimental fats are solid at room temperature, and their molecular shape and exceptional inflammatory nature make them particularly unhealthy. As my father used to say, "They gum up the works." In the cell membranes, they sabotage optimal function. Wherever they are, they incite inflammation.

Cutting out trans fats is part of the process that helps reduce joint pain, so do it now! (I'll show you how later in the book.) Your joints probably won't feel better as soon as tomorrow or the next day, but they definitely will feel better over time. And it won't be only your joints that feel better, either—reducing inflammation has a positive effect on all your body's systems.

Inside the Cell

The control center of the cell is the nucleus, by virtue of its DNA content. DNA, the director of the cell's actions, contains the plans or templates for all the molecules a cell can make, including those that will kick-start the inflammatory cycle.

Producing healthy, pain-preventing proteins (anti-inflammatory) and preventing the production of unhealthy, pain-causing proteins (inflammatory) are keys to joint health. For joints to feel better, the appropriate portion of DNA that codes for anti inflammatory proteins needs to be turned on, whereas the part coding for inflammatory proteins needs to stay off. I will show you how to influence the critical "caretaker" molecules that regulate the on and off switches of DNA.

Free radicals are a by-product of cell function that can damage cells and lead to inflammation. Antioxidants, because they neutralize free radicals and, therefore, inflammation, also play a role in preventing joint pain. Each day I spend a considerable amount of time explaining the benefits of antioxidants, so I understand all too well that many of my colleagues and patients doubt their benefits. If you are among those who doubt the benefits of antioxidants, review K. Yudoh's classic study in *Arthritis Research and Therapy* (2005), which definitively shows how free radicals ignite the molecular effects leading to osteoarthritis.

Antioxidants reverse pain-causing molecular effects. You can increase the number of antioxidants in your system by eating foods that are rich in these substances. This is just one more reason to eat your blueberries (among the many tasty antioxidants).

The Life and Death of Cells

Cells have life cycles, just like humans. Some people live long, healthy lives, while others are less fortunate and live shorter lives. Similarly, cells, depending on their function, have varying life spans. Nerve cells may last a lifetime, while red blood cells last 120 days, and white blood cells last only one day. The cell life cycle is coded in each cell's DNA. The cell cycle's final cascade of chemical events leading to cellular death is extremely important. Cell death occurs through apoptosis, where the cell essentially commits suicide when its preprogrammed time is up. This is important because we want old, failing cells to die before they promote inflammation or before their DNA mutates and turns cancerous. If cells don't die at their appointed times, they sometimes become immortal and grow out of control, first taking over an organ system and eventually the entire body. I bet you've never thought of cells becoming immortal, but that's what happens when a cell turns cancerous.

For the purpose of controlling joint pain, we are particularly concerned about maintaining the balance of inflammation of all the cells making up our joints. If we are to minimize joint pain, we must significantly influence the balance of the inflammatory seesaw. If cells need to die because their life cycle is over, then we need the process of cell death to occur cleanly and decisively so that no inflammation or, even worse, cancers occur.

Naturally, we also do not want healthy cells to die prematurely. We want the white blood cells supervising our joints to turn over daily and quickly, while tendon cells turn over only every several years. Cartilage is rather sparsely populated by cells, called chondrocytes. Imagine a bowl of Jell-O with a few pieces of fruit inside. That's like the structure of cartilage, Jell-O being the rubbery matrix and the few fruit pieces being the cells. Those few cells must maintain the health of the rubbery matrix of the cartilage, so keeping them healthy is quintessential to joint health. We don't want them to die too early, because they can't be replaced easily. Premature cartilage cell death leads to cartilage matrix breakdown, or arthritis.

Moreover, the significance of cell death goes way beyond joints. The same central regulatory linchpin that controls the production of the inflammatory molecules also influences the cell life cycle and can trigger disease in the joints, heart, or other organs. The fact that inflammation leads to disease in joints and many organs means that controlling inflammation can lead to joint health, as well as overall health. An anti-inflammatory lifestyle is an overall healthy lifestyle.

Ever wonder why we age or why we die? There's something called the inflammation hypothesis of aging, which states that cells age when the inflammatory cycle gets out of balance. As we get older, the inflammatory cycle becomes more active; this leads to cell-membrane, organelle, and DNA damage. Cell function and the normal cell cycle are disrupted. Cells that haven't reached their life expectancy die prematurely. Osteoarthritic joint pain results when inflammation impairs chondrocytes' function and when those cells die prematurely. Remember that chondrocytes are relatively few in number and have the massive responsibility of maintaining the rubbery, cushioning nature of joint cartilage. Losing too many chondrocytes prematurely leaves the cartilage structure at risk for joint arthritis and pain.

NUCLEAR FACTOR KAPPA BETA (NFkB)— THE NEXT BIG THING

The inflammatory pathways implicated in aging, arthritis, heart disease, cancer, and virtually every other disease process are at least partially controlled by a family of structurally similar molecules called nuclear factor kappa beta (NFkB). Joint pain involves several cell types: bone cells called osteoblasts and osteoclasts, joint-lining cells, white blood cells, and cartilage cells called chondrocytes. Each of these cells is on an inflammatory seesaw and is being pushed toward peace or pain by molecular messengers that I refer to as DNA "caretakers." Scientists refer to these "caretakers" as transcription factors. The chief caretaker that triggers the production of inflammatory molecules is NFkB.

The family of NFkB and its closely related transcription factors (NFkB, Nfat, SAF, SOX) will be the most intensely researched regulatory molecules that you will hear and read about in the next ten years. This group of molecules represents the DNA "caretakers" that we are specifically trying to influence to prevent joint pain. They are an extremely important and often sinister group, because they control the same inflammation that is implicated in many disease processes.

Some scientists have described NFkB as controlling the central pathway in the aging process. Because of this, it has an extraordinary influence on arthritis. One scientific article describes NFkB as the linchpin of inflammation-associated cancer (Li 2005). It is a controlling conspirator in heart disease, it's at the core of inflammatory bowel disease, and it is a central factor in joint pain.

NFkB was discovered in 1986 by Nobel Prize laureate David Baltimore. It's not one molecule, but a complex family of molecules that have the ability to influence DNA production of inflammatory proteins. They are responsible for the on switch for inflammation. If NFkB is active, it will jump-start the inflammatory cycle. When joint cells are stimulated by joint stresses, overuse, injury, or inflammatory foods, a cascade of events activates NFkBs. Any of the activated NFkB molecules can start the inflammatory process by triggering a chain of events. White blood cells, which produce inflammatory compounds, are summoned to the affected area. Blood vessels allow fluids to leak into the joint tissues. Pain-causing chemicals are released. The joint swells and hurts. Over time joint cartilage begins to degenerate. For joint-pain relief, it's vital to keep the NFkBs inactive. That's what my *Healthy Joints for Life* program does.

Caspase molecules are the "hit men" of the cell, killing the cell should it become damaged. When members of the NFkB family go into the nucleus, molecules that counteract caspases are formed. Without the caspases there is no way to eliminate damaged cells. If there's too much NFkB in a cell, a damaged, abnormal cell that should die isn't eliminated. That abnormal cell becomes immortal, and that leads to the uncontrolled replication of damaged cells. We call this cancer.

The *Healthy Joints for Life* program is based on identifying foods, supplements, and exercises (types and quantities) that will, among other things, help control the NFkB family of transcription factors or DNA caretakers. The identification of these foods, supplements, and exercises comes from scientific research published throughout the world. Over a decade ago, when I was introduced to the inflammatory concept of aging by forward-thinking doctors like Nick Perricone, M.D., and Stephen Sinatra, M.D., I immediately started thinking about joint pain and inflammation. I researched the chemical pathways of inflammation and started to go back to basics. I already understood the rationale and benefits of mainstream medicine, but slowly I started to see the benefits of a holistic approach and began to make suggestions to my patients. When NFkB was identified, I became fanatical about learning about its role in the inflammatory cascade. Hundreds of articles and countless patient interactions have given birth to this program.

Before we get to how you can make changes in your life that will have a dramatic effect on reducing your joint pain, we need to take a look at how a joint functions when it's healthy and what goes wrong when your joint's cells have run amok.

CHAPTER 2

JOINTS:
How They Work
and What Can Go Wrong

A JOINT IS A HINGE BETWEEN TWO BONES. THE ANATOMY OF some joints, like the hip and shoulder joints, allows a more encompassing range of motion, whereas others, like those of the fingers, "hinge" in only one plane. Joints allow the rigid adjacent bones to bend so that you can take a walk, throw a ball, pick up a pen off your desk, or engage in the many thousands of movements you do each day. Without the rigid structure of bones and the muscle units of the musculoskeletal system, we would not be upright or ambulatory. We would be like squid, lying in a heap. By virtue of our amazing joints and brilliantly designed musculoskeletal system, the wonders of locomotion and movement are possible. Life is motion.

In order for a joint to work at its best, it must be stable, smooth, and flexible. Stabilizing the ends of your bones is a tough, but flexible capsule made up of two layers. The inner lining of the capsule, called the synovium, produces nourishing and lubricating fluid. Its cellular components also play a major role in initiating inflammation and are currently the focus of significant research. The outer layer of the capsule is fibrous, tough, and strong. This layer comprises the ligaments of the joint, and their purpose is to firmly stabilize the joint by connecting and aligning the bones.

To allow for near frictionless motion and to provide cushioning, the ends of the bones are covered with smooth articular cartilage. The rubbery articular cartilage cushions the ends of the bones, while the synovial fluid, secreted by the synovium, lubricates and nourishes the smooth articular surfaces. When joints are in correct alignment, the smooth bony ends glide against one another virtually without friction.

Articular cartilage is a highly specialized tissue. It is composed of cartilage cells, called chondrocytes, which produce a matrix that gives cartilage its rubbery nature. Older theories on osteoarthritis concentrated on the breakdown of cartilage from mechanical stresses, like increased body weight or trauma or injury. *Healthy Joints for Life* will show you how the molecular action of inflammation provides a less obvious, but considerable cause for cartilage and joint degradation. Joints with less cushion ultimately become painful.

State-of-the-art theory on joint degeneration indicates that synovium, bone, and cartilage all play interrelated roles in the degenerative process. The synovium swells and delivers inflammatory cells to the joint. Cartilage matrix production and degradation get out of balance, resulting in articular cartilage loss. As the cushioning of the articular cartilage is lost, the bone has no choice but to absorb more mechanical stresses. And as the bone absorbs those forces, it attempts to fortify itself, but in the process it ends up growing abnormally. The bone's abnormal attempts at strengthening actually lead to a contradictory weakening and collapse. Sinister molecules with erosive intentions bathe the bone and cartilage. Blood flow to the bone lessens. Like a death spiral, the weakened bone negatively impacts the articular cartilage and vice versa. This devious process, which leads to joint pain and swelling, is known as osteoarthritis. This is primarily the type of arthritis that we are fighting in this book.

There are more than one hundred types of arthritis. They include rheumatoid, psoriatic, infectious, and neuropathic arthritis. The most common variety, however, is osteoarthritis, otherwise known as classic "wear and tear" arthritis. But we are learning that osteoarthritis involves much more than just wear and tear. My mother had a very common arthritis, one sometimes confused with osteoarthritis, called rheumatoid arthritis (RA). This is a completely different disease than osteoarthritis, with a distinctly different cause. RA is an autoimmune arthritis where the patient's immune system malfunctions and joint cells are misidentified as the enemy and are mistakenly attacked by the patient's own immune system. Osteoarthritis is not an autoimmune disease. It can be caused by wear and tear, but it is also a disease of out-of-control inflammation.

INFLAMMATION AND YOUR JOINTS

Inflammation starts its attack at the molecular level, directly influencing cellular function and, ultimately, anatomic joint structures. By understanding inflammation and the basics of how the joints work, we can formulate a plan to fight joint pain.

For our purposes, we don't need to learn all the nuances of joint structure, but we do need to learn the basic concepts so that we can understand how joints become painful. The image I'd like you to remember is the following clean, clear-cut, simplified diagram, which shows all the important structures of the knee joint.

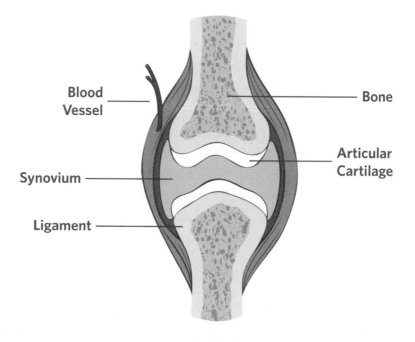

Blood Vessel

Bone

Synovium

Articular Cartilage

Ligament

THE SYNOVIAL JOINT

The synovial joint is formed where the ends of two bones meet. The total thickness of the articular cartilage that covers the ends of bones varies, but it can be nearly one centimeter thick in some weight-bearing joints, like the knee and hip. The articular surface cushions the bones and helps absorb stress. In the case of a weight-bearing joint, like the knee, large amounts of stress are absorbed in simple activities like walking, running, or jumping. In the case of non-weight-bearing joints, like the fingers, smaller quantities of stress are absorbed.

LIGAMENTS

A ligament is a band of tissue that serves as a connection between bones. The capsule depicted in the following diagram of the hip joint surrounds the smooth rubbery ends of the bones. The tough outer fibrous portion of this capsule connects and stabilizes the two bony ends. These thickened areas of the fibrous capsule are commonly known as the ligaments of the joint.

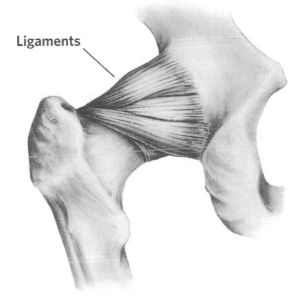

Ligaments

Maintaining a healthy articular surface depends on having strong, firm ligaments. A torn ligament leads to a wobbly, unstable joint with asymmetrical or uneven rubbing of the articular cartilage and premature wear of the joint. Think about how the bottom of a shoe wears. If you walk solely on the outer portion of the heel, it will wear out on that side. If you walk in a neutral position, the load across the whole heel is shared, and the heel will last longer. Similarly, ligaments keep joints in a neutral position and allow the joints to last longer.

MY LIFE'S DEDICATION

A sports-related torn anterior cruciate ligament (ACL) may be the quintessential example of how a torn ligament can lead to an arthritic joint. The ACL is a small but critical stabilizing ligament in the central portion of the knee. It is

continued

about 1½ inches long and ⅜ inch thick, yet it has an incredible effect on joint health. When it is torn or damaged the knee buckles, and the instability of the knee can lead to other injuries on the inside of the knee, like meniscal cartilage tears. Studies show that ACL-deficient knees become arthritic over decades. Healthy knees of people with intact ACLs (who are the same age as people with ACL-deficient knees) do not degenerate at anywhere near the same rate.

As a practicing knee and shoulder surgeon, I have dedicated a large portion of my life to reconstructing that little but essential ligament.

SYNOVIUM

The inner membrane of the capsule, the synovium, is paper-thin. It is the layer that produces the synovial fluid and forms a thin barrier that allows the flow of fluid and molecules in and out of the joint. If bacteria is around a joint, then the body sends messengers to bring in white blood cells to defend against infection. As a result, necessary helpful inflammation occurs, but we don't want any more inflammation than is absolutely required. Unfortunately, our lifestyles are leading to *unnecessary* inflammation. If you eat a lot of trans fats, saturated fats, or omega-6 fats, then the cell membranes of cells of the synovium will become populated with molecules that can call for inflammation. It's a different mechanism than the cells' response to invading bacteria, but it has the same end result—inflammation. If you eat poorly, smoke, and drink too much alcohol, you will produce too many damaging charged particles called free radicals, which injure your cells and cause inflammation. Your joints will swell and hurt.

Inflammation is a normal process, but when it gets out of control, it causes damage to the joints and the body. The inflammation beginning in the cells of the synovium is at the center of the state-of-the-art scientific movement to define osteoarthritis as a "whole joint" disease, rather than one solely involving the cartilage of the joints. The program in this book will help to curtail unnecessary inflammation, which can cause pain. The NFkB family of DNA caretakers is a key mediator of this process, and that's why we are trying to control it through diet, exercise, and supplements.

SYNOVIAL FLUID

The synovial fluid has a dual purpose. It lubricates the joint surfaces, and because the articular cartilage is not vascularized, meaning it has no blood vessels coursing through it, the synovial fluid also provides the articular cartilage surface with nutrients, such as glucose and proteins/amino acids. (Strings of amino acids make up proteins.)

Some amino acids in the synovial fluid float around individually, while others are strung together to form proteins. Synovial fluid is composed of hyaluronate (hyaluronate is also sometimes referred to as hyaluronic acid and hyaluronan), lubricin, proteinases (enzymes that breakdown proteins), and collagenases (enzymes that breakdown collagen). This fluid can cushion (hyaluronan), lubricate (lubricin), and play a part in the body's constant breakdown (proteinases, collagenases) and replenishment of the joint surface.

Hyaluronate is made of D-glucuronic acid and D-N-acetyl-glucosamine. You have probably heard that many people take glucosamine as a supplement, and now you know part of the reason why: it is a building block for the synovial fluid component hyaluronate, sort of like WD-40 for joints. It is an important molecule that is also part of the matrix, or "Jell-O-like" portion, of cartilage, which I mentioned earlier.

Too much synovial fluid, generated in reaction to irritation of the joint, can bathe the articular cartilage in a rather caustic blend of enzymes (proteinases and collagenases), breaking down the cartilage over time.

When a joint becomes arthritic, the articular cartilage breaks down, but that is not the only thing that happens. While the old theory on osteoarthritis centered on the damage that occurs in articular cartilage, current research has expanded the theory to include articular cartilage in combination with bones, white blood cells, and synovium. Clearly, there is a cascade of events involving the synovium, white blood cells, bone, and articular cartilage. Like falling dominos, they all play a role in the development of osteoarthritis.

Joint pain can also come from injuries ranging from mild to severe. Simple overuse can cause the irritation of joint components—the capsule, the synovium, articular cartilage, or even bone. Irritation starts the cascade of inflammation, with increased permeability of blood vessels, leading to swelling, or edema. White blood cells leak into the tissue, secreting inflammation-provoking cytokine messengers, which directly or indirectly lead to pain. With sufficient injury, small blood vessels may tear, leading to bleeding into the joint. To control the bleeding, a host of clotting factors are secreted. Within moments the joint becomes swollen and painful.

In the inflammatory process, cells that line the walls of blood vessels, called endothelial cells, actually spread apart, so that blood plasma fluid and even white blood cells leak into the joint capsule.

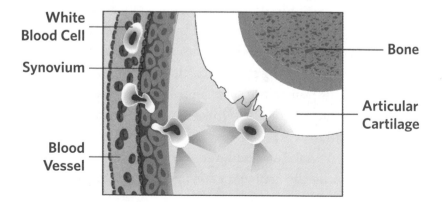

White blood cells, in their quest to patrol the joint for infectious invaders, can secrete damaging free radicals, which injure healthy tissue. Like in a war, collateral damage occurs, and innocent joint cells, whether they be cartilage, ligament, or bone, sustain cellular damage. As the nerve endings sense tissue damage and swelling, they send pain messages via small molecules, like substance P, a protein messenger, to the brain. Through the autonomic nervous system, blood flow to the joint increases, sending additional nourishment to help, but additional fluid arrives as well, causing more swelling. The joint begins to hurt.

ARTICULAR CARTILAGE

Articular cartilage covers and cushions the ends of the bones. Water is a key component to maintaining the flexibility and health of articular cartilage, and it represents up to 87 percent of articular cartilage weight. As we age, sugar proteins in joint cartilage decrease, and because these molecules harbor water, the water content of joint cartilage is reduced, as well. This leads to a decrease in the "rubberiness" of the articular cartilage. Cartilage becoming "brittle" is an important characteristic of osteoarthritis.

Interspersed with the water retaining sugar proteins are collagen molecules. Collagen and sugar proteins form the rubbery matrix superstructure of the articular cartilage. Collagen is an extremely important component of cartilage, representing two-thirds of dry cartilage weight. While the amazing DNA that directs each and every cell in the body has a fascinating two-limbed helix structure, the collagen of the joints is even more intricate, as it is a triple-limbed helix (like a braid) of amino acids. Located throughout the bone's cap, the collagen of articular cartilage is specifically arranged into three layers based on the depth and orientation of the collagen fibers.

The fibers' orientation defines the function of the layer. In the outermost, superficial layer the collagen is parallel to the joint surface, providing tensile strength, which doesn't cushion but keeps the layers from shearing off under stress. This outer layer is like the leather upholstery on a car seat, which protects the cushion beneath. It is difficult to break through this outer layer of collagen, but just like the leather on your car seat, once that layer is breached, the next layers break down more easily. As soon as the leather upholstery wears through, the foam cushion will begin to disintegrate. Similarly, the next two layers in cartilage disintegrate quickly, as their fiber orientation does not fight shear. Of the three layers of collagen, the middle layer provides cushioning via its random collagen orientation, while the layer closest to the bone has a perpendicular orientation, which attaches the cartilage to the bone.

Joint Articular Cartilage Surface

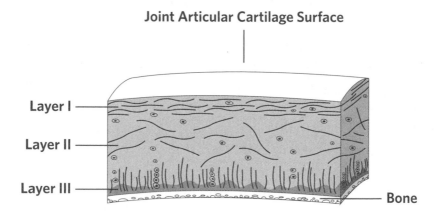

Layer I

Layer II

Layer III

Bone

Chondrocytes are living cells that have the ability to make collagen and glycosaminoglycans (GAGs), just like a cell of the pancreas can make insulin. Because cartilage is avascular, meaning that blood vessels do not penetrate the matrix, nutrients that the chondrocytes need must seep into the cartilage structure through a process called diffusion. The synovial fluid, which bathes the cartilage, provides nutrients, as well as lubrication. Nutrients can also diffuse into the articular cartilage from the area where the bone and cartilage meet. That is where bone marrow nutrients diffuse or seep into the cartilage.

CARTILAGE AND JOINT HEALTH

Healthy cartilage is maintained by a healthy balance of matrix synthesis and degradation. Degradation is a natural part of the process. As particles age and deform, we want them replaced. It is similar to the way your skin cells are shed and replaced. The collagen must be maintained for tensile strength, while the sugar proteins must be maintained for their ability to capture water and provide cushioning. The chondrocytes are required to maintain the balance of this essential process. You can support the function of the chondrocytes through nutrition, exercise, and supplements.

DYNAMIC VERSUS STATIC COMPRESSION OF JOINTS

The dynamic compression of joints and the static compression of joints are important concepts in understanding how to maintain articular cartilage health. Dynamic compression happens when the joint is squeezed together while moving, and static compression occurs when the joint is squeezed while not in motion. Walking is an example of dynamic compression, while kneeling is an example of static compression. Dynamic compression of the joint is quite healthy for the balance of cartilage matrix production, and simple physics explains why static compression is harder on your joints. Cartilage is better at absorbing forces than dissipating forces, and because the force can't come out as easily as it goes in (via impact on the joint), the cartilage may crack to release the energy (Fulcher 2009).

Think about kids jumping up and down on a trampoline. The higher up they go in the air, the more force they come down with and then the higher up they go again. Well, cartilage is not a perfect trampoline. It doesn't return all the energy applied to it. Instead, some of the force is absorbed by the cartilage itself. If too much is absorbed, then the cartilage will literally explode or crack to relieve the stress. If the joint is moving, then the force is spread over a bigger area, and that keeps the cartilage from becoming damaged. With static compression, the force is exerted in one place for an extended amount of time, and there is very little release of pressure or force. This is part of the reason why people who work on their knees, such as carpet layers, often develop arthritis.

It's also important to know that motion, all by itself, is healthy because it stimulates the synovium to produce synovial fluid. Healthy articular cartilage is nice and smooth (image on the left), but the slippery synovial fluid makes those nice smooth surfaces move with virtually no friction. Degenerative articular cartilage that is actively breaking down can be seen on the right in the following diagram.

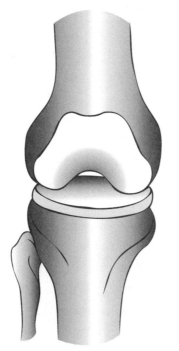 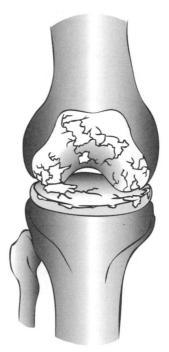

THE NFL AND JOINT PAIN

NFL players are paid to play football, and many times that means disregarding painful, swollen joints. All of us who played professionally played in pain—including me. What happens over time when you disregard painful, swollen joints? It's no secret that many of my teammates are suffering terribly after years of neglecting and abusing their joints. As a former player and an orthopedic surgeon, I understand that joint injury is a part of the game of football that few avoid. Despite extraordinary talents and body awareness, no NFL player is spared from the traumas that lead to osteoarthritis. In fact, you don't have to be an NFL player to be subject to the forces that give rise to osteoarthritis. No one is spared, not me, you, or anyone else you know. We all wear out; it's just that some of us do things that accelerate the process.

Most of my teammates will admit that some of their joints really hurt, and they can also point to countless games where they played hurt. Some can even tell you which NFL game led to their current pains. "That 49ers game on the turf got my left knee" or "That Patriots game we played in the snow nailed my right."

I can tell you that my teammates were dedicated, tough men. They gave a large part of their lives and numerous healthy body parts to the game, and joint pain is their uncompromising, unceasing reminder of how hard they played. The exhilaration of playing football is addicting, but there is a price to be paid for the fix. I'd bet most of my teammates wouldn't trade the experience for just about anything, but some are still suffering for the honor and the opportunity.

UNCHECKED INFLAMMATION

If inflammation proceeds unchecked, like a spark plug that never stops sparking, the joint becomes chronically swollen, and the articular surface is bathed in caustic fluids. The NFkB family gets activated from multiple stimuli. Collagen starts to degrade, and water is lost through the deterioration of sugar-protein molecules called GAGs. The cartilage cells can't maintain the delicate and essential synthesis/degradation balance. The articular surface goes from smooth to rough and/or cracked. Articular cartilage loses its ability to cushion. Cartilage cells start to die.

As the articular cartilage breaks down, it loses its mechanical integrity and its cushioning ability. Its ability to store energy decreases, and impacts that were previously well tolerated cause cracks in the surfaces. Soon millions of minute particles of articular cartilage— cartilage sawdust—are irritating the synovium. These particles increase NFkB production, along with other inflammatory agents. A vicious cycle starts, with increased production of synovial fluid full of degrading enzymes, further cartilage breakdown, and additional pain and swelling of the joint. Inflammation proceeds unchecked.

INFLAMMATION AND CARTILAGE DEGENERATION

Overload on the joints (both active and static) can cause cartilage degradation, but our old nemesis inflammation also leads to cartilage breaking down, which in turn gives rise to joint pain and problems. Other disease processes, like rheumatoid arthritis, lead to a breakdown in cartilage but through different mechanisms. Typically, the Jell-O-like extracellular matrix (ECM) of cartilage turns over slowly. The sugar proteins and collagen molecules making up the matrix last a long time, that is, until inflammation takes over.

With pro-inflammatory stimuli, the cartilage cells (embedded in the cartilage Jell-O-like ECM) and/or the synovial cells (in the knee lining or synovium) produce inflammatory cytokine molecules. Those inflammatory molecules are like battery acid, breaking down the sugar proteins and collagen. Inflammatory stimuli affect all the components of the joint, so, for example, bone, white blood cells, cartilage cells, or synovial cells can produce inflammatory molecules that degrade the Jell-O-like ECM. Out-of-balance, exaggerated inflammation leads to degradation. When the production of new ECM can't keep up with the degradation, then the cartilage breaks down and loses its cushioning ability.

Similarly, synovial cells can make too much synovial fluid, which is teeming with the proteinases and collagenases that bathe the cartilage and degrade the matrix, as well. That excessive synovial fluid represents what is commonly known as "water on the knee."

MATRIX METALLOPROTEINASES (MMPs)—
THE MOLECULES THAT DEGRADE COLLAGEN

Perhaps the most destructive cytokine inflammatory molecules (molecules secreted by cells that communicate with and alter other cell functions) of all the cytokines that DNA caretaker NFkB and closely related caretaker AP-1 (activator protein-1) control are matrix metalloproteinases (MMPs). They are so terribly destructive, in fact, that I feel that they are molecular public enemy number one. These enzymes are like battery acid to ECM. Single-handedly they can break down ECM and, in particular, collagen. The worst of the MMPs, numbers 1 and 13, are so corrosive to collagen that they are called collagenase 1 and 3. As the term collagenase implies, these enzymes break down collagen, robbing the cartilage of much of its strength. It is extremely important to block AP-1 and NFkBs in order to prevent the production of MMPs.

AGGRECANASES—THE MOLECULES
THAT DEGRADE SUGAR PROTEINS

Sugar proteins are not ignored when it comes to cartilage degradation. Enzymes called aggrecanases, also produced under the regulation of DNA caretakers AP-1 and NFkB, will break down sugar proteins. Recall that the branched structure of sugar proteins retains water molecules, which give cartilage its wonderful rubbery structure. As sugar proteins break down, water is lost and so is the cushioning effect of cartilage.

NITRIC OXIDE

Nitric oxide (NO) is a molecule that impacts many tissues throughout the body. Some of its effects are beneficial; others are detrimental. For example, nitric oxide is extremely beneficial for the cardiovascular system. It facilitates blood vessel endothelial cell health, while increasing blood flow through vessels by relaxing the smooth muscle cells of vessel walls. Nitric oxide's effect on articular cartilage, however, leads to extensive chondrocyte damage. We, therefore, want nitric oxide for vessel health but not for cartilage health. Maintaining a balance of NO allows us to preserve the benefits to the cardiovascular system while keeping the potential for joint damage in check. Too much nitric oxide will tip the chondrocyte production/degradation balance in the wrong direction, leading to osteoarthritis and joint pain. Decreasing levels of free radicals by means of joint-healthy supplements and an optimal diet keeps NO levels in check.

ADVANCED GLYCATION END PRODUCTS (AGEs)

Advanced glycation end products (AGEs) occur when sugars stick to the collagen of cartilage or ligaments, causing "aging" or stiffening of those structures. The acronym AGEs reinforces the idea that the process literally "ages" the joint. If sugar levels are persistently high, like in those with diabetes or those who have terrible diets, then cartilage and ligament aging is more likely to occur. The joint becomes stiff and brittle.

WHEN THE JOB SEEMS INSURMOUNTABLE

Football at the NFL level is a game of survival. Being able to maintain your composure with maniacs running all around you is no easy job. My more civilized friends might call it "downright alarming." It's important to try to slow things down, stay poised, and use your intelligence along with your brawn. Sometimes it works; sometimes it doesn't.

My most memorable kickoff return came against the Baltimore Colts—and I didn't even carry the ball. At the beginning of the 1982 preseason I was the return man directly to the right of the primary deep return man, Fulton Walker. Depending on where the ball was kicked there was a good chance I could be the ballcarrier. As the season progressed we developed some blocking problems and, to my chagrin, I was "elevated" to captain of the wedge—the middle man of the three-man blocking wedge formed directly in front of the ball-carrying return man—with 285-pound bookends Cleveland Green and Roy Foster to my left and right. I asked special-teams coach Steve Crosby what I was doing between those two behemoths, and he said, "Shula said he needed a smart, crazy SOB to lead the wedge. He meant you." He might have been pulling my chain, or he was thinking I was expendable, but I took it as the ultimate compliment.

When the ball was kicked, my job as captain of the wedge was to drop the three-man wedge to about twelve yards in front of the ballcarrier. When the ballcarrier caught the ball, I yelled, "Go!" and we would charge upfield, blocking in unison any kamikaze coverage guys. Sometimes we would be assigned specific guys to block—and that's exactly what I was assigned to do against the Colts. The problem was that the six-foot-two, 235-pound linebacker who was on the pregame scouting sheets was hurt, replaced by a six-foot-seven, 270-pound defensive lineman. As I reviewed my assignment, I quickly noted that I had to block Herman Munster running at full speed, and he would crush me if I took him straight on.

I quickly formulated a plan to hide in the confusion off to the right and then blindside him at the last second. The plan worked beautifully until that last second, when he saw me coming. The collision was incredible. His forearm smashed into my face mask, twisting my head ninety degrees and nearly ripping my helmet off. My cleats flew from underneath me, the sky spinning, clouds whirling. I bounced on the ground a few times before settling beneath the grunting obscenities of the giant.

"#@$%, you try that again and I'll knock your head clean off and eat it."

I could only mumble, "You eat my head, and you'll have more brains in your stomach than in your own head."

On the next kickoff Coach Crosby mercifully reassigned me to block another guy. He said with a smile, "Rich, I'm going to change your blocking assignment. I don't want that guy to break his arm on your head."

OSTEOARTHRITIS

Earlier in this chapter I told you that osteoarthritis, often referred to as "wear and tear" arthritis, is caused by mechanical wear and tear, as well as molecular factors. I used the analogy of the shoe sole wearing down unevenly. On the surface it's a good analogy, but in order to make it more accurate, we need to add to it. Imagine that the surface you are walking on is coated with acid, so that the acid eats away at the sole at the same time that the sole sustains surface wear from use. That more accurately portrays the mechanical and inflammatory impact on joints that leads to the breakdown of the components of articular cartilage.

WHAT HAPPENS TO THE BONE
WHEN INFLAMMATION IS LEFT UNCHECKED?

As the cushioning of the cartilaginous articular surface lessens, the bone absorbs more of the impact from activities. Sensing greater mechanical forces, the bone reacts by growing and attempting to strengthen itself. The inflamed synovial lining cells migrate onto the corners of the bone. A barrage of deleterious molecular messages is also sent to the bone. The blood flow to the bone lessens, decreasing the nourishment for the bone itself, as well as for the cartilage overlying it.

The capsule, composed of the thin, membranous synovium and the thick, fibrous ligaments, is attached to and firmly connects the ends of the two bones of a joint. The capsule fully surrounds the joint so that it is watertight and will contain the synovial fluid that lubricates the articular cartilage surfaces. As the articular cartilage thins, the bone feels more stress, and the synovium attachment sites are altered, with synovium growing toward the articular cartilage edge.

The problem is twofold: the synovium's abnormal migration to the edge of the articular cartilage, in combination with the bone's misguided attempt at fortifying itself, actually leads to the inappropriate formation of bone spurs—pointy pieces of bone on the bone edge—and the unintentional weakening of bone. When bone is resorbed and therefore weakened, the lack of strong underlying bone causes the cartilage to sag and crack. Furthermore, blood flow to the weakened bone diminishes, lessening the natural flow of nourishment to the cartilage.

Ultimately, range of motion is lost, and muscles weaken. Acting as a "volume switch" the nervous system attempts to protect the joint by reducing muscle stimulation. Messages sent from the swollen, painful joint cause a reflex spinal cord response, decreasing nerve impulses and therefore muscle strength.

Consider what happened when the knee of a caveman or cave-woman was hurt. Cave people were *capa tosta*, as my grandma Bellucci would say, "thickheaded," so it was important that the body protect itself. The knee swelled and the body automatically decreased its muscle strength so the cave person literally couldn't keep running after the woolly mammoth or saber-toothed tiger he or she was trying to kill. The weakened muscle forced the cave person to rest.

NFkB plays a primary role in the weakening of bone by misleading bone-forming and bone-resorbing cells. Meanwhile, NFkB's DNA caretaker cousin SAF-1 plays a primary role in the formation of joint-deforming bone spurs.

In attempting to preserve the joint, the body is making an effort to protect itself from ruination. Decreased nerve stimulation translates into muscle weakness. The painful, swollen, severely arthritic joint succumbs to a restricted range of motion and muscle weakness. Once you have irreversibly severe joint disease (once it is so bad that no medicine or program such as mine will help), joint replacement is the most effective treatment.

The following sequence of pictures shows:

❶ An X-ray of severe knee arthritis.
❷ A postoperative X-ray of the knee replacement in place.

This book will not change the fact that severe joint disease is irreversible and terribly painful. Surgery, in such cases, is most likely necessary. For those who cannot have surgery, all is not lost. We may not be able to reverse the arthritis, but we may be able to deliver some joint-pain relief, even in quite difficult situations.

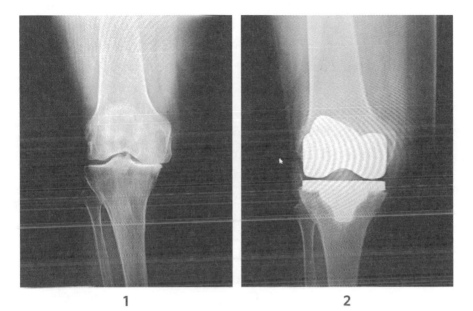

1   2

Clearly, joint replacement is the last resort treatment for end-stage osteoarthritis. Most people are not at the end stage, and even those with moderately severe joint disease can obtain some relief from pain by halting the inflammatory cycle.

WHAT CAN WE DO?

By understanding the mechanical and molecular processes that are occurring in joints, we now have the groundwork to determine how to stop the inflammation and the pain of arthritis, which usually lands you in the office of an orthopedic surgeon, sometimes directly or sometimes through your medical doctor. If it is determined that you have a mild or moderate degree of osteoarthritis, you are typically prescribed nonsteroidal anti-inflammatories (Motrin, Naprosyn, Mobic, Celebrex) or perhaps given an injection of cortisone or lubricants (Synvisc, Orthovisc). Sometimes braces or orthotics might be recommended. If the osteoarthritis is severe enough, then surgery may be the most appropriate treatment. However, surgery is the last resort. Yes, you read that correctly, and it is directly from an orthopedic surgeon. Surgery is the last resort. For those who are willing to take a more proactive part in their care, there may be other options, even for those with relatively severe osteoarthritis.

There are things we can do to help control the inflammatory process at the heart of osteoarthritic pain. We know what causes inflammation and what can go wrong in the knee and other joints due to injury, impact, or overuse. We need to knock out each of these inciting elements. We need to stop the process in its tracks early. If the train is already halfway there, we must keep it from going any farther. We need to stop inflammation and modify joint stresses. We need to stop, or at least slow, the degradation of the joint. Because we know how the joint is being degraded, mechanically and molecularly, we can attempt to control those elements and block those pathways. I can show you how to control joint stresses and inflammation with diet, supplements, and exercise. Let's get started.

CHAPTER 3

EAT:
Foods That Reduce Joint Pain

SOME OF THE FOODS WE EAT ARE NUTRITIOUS, AND SOME ARE absolutely delicious. Some embody our traditions and heritage. But not all are especially kind to our joints. I am going to help you to make better choices when it comes to the foods you eat. What you eat can have a major impact on how your joints feel. The scientific research on foods that combat inflammation is growing quickly. The foods I am going to recommend to you will combat inflammation, reduce joint pain, and even help you to reduce your weight. These foods will be the ones you select to create your eating plan through-out the eight weeks of the program—and beyond. Eating is impor-tant for many reasons. Let's add reducing joint pain to that list.

THE ELEVEN NUTRITIONAL COMMANDMENTS FOR JOINT HEALTH

❶ Thou shall respect insulin as the body's primary inflammatory hormone and recognize that it is secreted in direct response to eating carbohydrates.

❷ Thou shall control blood sugar levels by understanding the glycemic index and load of specific carbohydrates and by eating slower-digesting complex carbohydrates.

3 Thou shall help control blood sugar levels with fiber.

4 Thou shall avoid high fructose corn syrup.

5 Thou shall avoid trans fats.

6 Thou shall eat "smart" saturated fats, minimize processed polyunsaturated fats, and beware of fried foods, especially those fried in polyunsaturated fats.

7 Thou shall maximize omega-3 fatty acids.

8 Thou shall remember that omega-6 fatty acids are unsaturated and essential but still need to be minimized, because they are so easily oxidized and are the basis for inflammatory pathway building block, arachidonic acid.

9 Thou shall eat as much fish as possible, keeping in mind that salmon is preferable to all others.

10 Thou shall choose healthier animal proteins, like buffalo, chicken, and turkey, and leaner cuts of those proteins, like the strip and breast.

The Bonus Commandment:

11 Thou shall combine healthy fats and proteins with healthy carbohydrates in order to effectively reduce the glycemic index (GI) of the carbohydrates.

The types of carbohydrates, fats, and proteins we choose to eat can have a dramatic effect on how our joints feel. You can control inflammation and joint pain by eating joint-healthy foods. Sorting out which foods are beneficial to joint health is fairly easy as we eat only three categories of foods, namely, carbohydrates, fats, and proteins. That's basically it.

You can get picky and debate where to put alcohol or sugar alcohols, but for our purposes it's worth reemphasizing that if you eat it, then it's a carbohydrate, fat, or protein. I often refer to those food groups as The Big Three. If you learn to balance The Big Three you will be one step closer to controlling joint pain.

CARBOHYDRATES

Carbohydrates are broken down into glucose (aka blood sugar) by the body, and insulin is secreted in response to glucose. Both glucose and insulin are inflammatory and, in excess, can be damaging to our joints. Carbohydrate consumption needs to be monitored closely, or else inflammation will ensue. I believe that carbohydrates are the most underestimated and misunderstood of The Big Three. I say that because their systemic inflammatory effects are so extensive. I don't want to demonize carbohydrates in the way that fats have sometimes been demonized. The fact is that some fats are very healthy, and many carbohydrates are, as well. What I will show you is which carbohydrates are joint friendly and which you would be better off avoiding.

You may be surprised to learn that bread, pasta, broccoli, and gummy worms are all carbohydrates. When I point out to patients that gummy worms and broccoli are both carbohydrates, they are usually skeptical. A typical response is, "You're kidding me, right?" By their expressions, I know most think I'm nuts (which, by the way, contain carbs, too). The fact remains that broccoli and gummy worms are not nutritional equivalents, but both are carbohydrates. The body digests them as carbohydrates.

DIGESTION 101

The way your body processes the foods you eat is an important part of understanding how your body uses nutrients. Carbohydrates are digested into the basic sugars, most

continued

important, glucose. Proteins are digested into amino acids. Fats are digested primarily into free fatty acids. Carbohydrates are an important energy source that provides quick energy, but they are not as energy dense as fat (carbs have four calories per gram, and fat has nine calories per gram). Fat is an important energy source and is the form in which energy is stored for the long term. Fat is also important for cell membrane formation and hormone formation (one of cholesterol's roles). Amino acids form the body's proteins, which are important for organ structure, like muscles and bone, but are also the basis of cellular communication, as they serve as the chemical messengers transmitting signals and information from one cell to another.

Many foods that are carbohydrates contain other nutrients, as well, including vitamins, which impact a carbohydrate's health and nutritional value. For the moment, I am going to concentrate on carbohydrate metabolism—how your body converts carbohydrates into energy. Later I'll discuss the other nutrients that are often found alongside carbohydrates and their impact on joint health.

FIBER

Fiber is a carbohydrate that the body cannot metabolize. It is very joint healthy, as well as being a digestive aid. Fiber's structure classifies it as a carbohydrate. Because our enzymes can't digest it, it has no caloric value. Fiber is one of nature's gifts to us all—no calories, aids digestion, and adds to our feeling full! There are two types of fiber—soluble and insoluble. Both should be included in your daily diet, because they are very joint friendly and have additional health benefits!

Soluble fiber is found in fruits, such as prunes, berries, and bananas, and in vegetables, such as peas, broccoli, carrots, onions, and sweet potatoes. It is also in grains, like oats and barley, as well as legumes (beans). Soluble fiber is distinguished by its ability to dissolve in water. It is fermented in the intestines by the normal intestinal bacteria that live and grow there. Soluble fiber can slow down glucose absorption, thereby helping to regulate blood glucose levels. When fiber is fermented by bacteria, short-chain fatty acids are formed. These have multiple health benefits, including managing glucose levels, suppressing total cholesterol and LDL "bad" cholesterol production, and improving the lining of the colon, which is so important for water and food absorption.

Insoluble fiber is not soluble in water. It is not fermented in the colon. It can't be digested or absorbed and therefore just adds bulk, which makes elimination easier. It also speeds the passage of food through the digestive tract. Whole grains, wheat, bran, nuts, seeds, tomato skins, green beans, cauliflower, and zucchini all contain insoluble fiber. Fruits like bananas and prunes contain both soluble and insoluble fiber.

Soluble fiber's ability to slow carbohydrate absorption and reduce blood sugar levels is very important for maintaining inflammatory balance. Soluble fiber forms a gel in the stomach, slowing down the passage of food out of the stomach and thereby making you feel full. Insoluble fiber increases bulk in the intestine and speeds things along. Soluble fiber lowers cholesterol, and insoluble fiber's influence on food transit keeps us regular and happy. Everyone should consume both soluble and insoluble fiber.

Various studies indicate that soluble and insoluble fiber have a significant anti-inflammatory effect on circulating cytokines in general, as well as specific inflammation. It is felt that fiber increases glucose sensitivity and helps impede fat absorption, so it can be beneficial for weight loss, too. The recommended amount of fiber is about .15 grams per pound of body weight. For a 200-pound person, that works out to thirty grams per day; for a 135-pound person, it would be twenty grams per day.

Consuming the correct amount of fiber daily will have wonderful effects on your digestion and food absorption. It will favorably influence sugar levels and help battle inflammation. By keeping your sugar levels down, your insulin level will be lowered and therefore will have a direct and subduing effect on the inflammation conductor NFkB. As a bonus, fiber makes you feel full, so it's a great component of a weight-loss program. The foods I mentioned above as examples of soluble and insoluble fiber are all full of fiber, but you could consider taking a daily fiber supplement to ensure hitting your target numbers. The table below, adapted from commonsensehealth.com, will point you in the right direction.

HIGH FIBER FOODS

(The fiber count for most packaged foods can be found on the nutrition label.)

FRUIT	AMOUNT	FIBER (grams)
Apples with skin	1 medium	5.0
Apricots	3 medium	1.0
Apricots, dried	5 pieces	2.9
Bananas	1 medium	3.9
Blueberries	1 cup	4.2
Cantaloupe, cubes	1 cup	1.3
Figs, dried	2 medium	3.7
Grapefruit	½ medium	3.1
Oranges, navel	1 medium	3.4
Peaches	1 medium	2.0
Peaches, dried	3 pieces	3.2
Pears	1 medium	5.1

FRUIT	AMOUNT	FIBER (grams)
Plums	1 medium	1.1
Raisins	1.5 oz box	1.6
Raspberries	1 cup	6.4 -
Strawberries	1 cup	4.4

VEGETABLES	AMOUNT	FIBER (grams)
Avocados (fruit)	1 medium	11.8 •
Bok choy, cooked	1 cup	2.8
Broccoli, cooked	1 cup	4.5 •
Brussels sprouts	1 cup	3.6
Cabbage, cooked	1 cup	4.2
Cauliflower, cooked	1 cup	3.4
Cole slaw	1 cup	4.0
Collard greens, cooked	1 cup	2.6
Green beans	1 cup	4.0 •
Celery	1 stalk	1.0
Kale, cooked	1 cup	7.2 •
Onions, raw	1 cup	2.9
Peas, cooked	1 cup	8.8 •
Peppers, sweet	1 cup	2.6
Popcorn, air-popped	3 cups	3.6
Potatoes, baked with skin	1 medium	4.8
Spinach, cooked	1 cup	4.3
Summer squash, cooked	1 cup	2.5
Sweet potatoes, cooked	1 cup	4.9 •
Swiss chard, cooked	1 cup	3.7
Tomatoes	1 medium	1.0
Winter squash, cooked	1 cup	6.2 •
Zucchini, cooked	1 cup	2.6

continued

CEREAL, GRAINS, PASTA	AMOUNT	FIBER (grams)
Bran cereal	1 cup	19.9
Bread, whole wheat	1 slice	2.0
Oats, rolled, dry	1 cup	12.0
Pasta, whole wheat	1 cup	6.3
Rice, dry brown	1 cup	8.0
BEANS, NUTS, SEEDS	**AMOUNT**	**FIBER (grams)**
Almonds	1 oz	4.2
Black beans, cooked	1 cup	14.9
Cashews	1 oz	1.0
Flaxseeds	3 tbs	7.0
Garbanzo beans, cooked	1 cup	5.8
Kidney beans, cooked	1 cup	13.3
Lentils, red, cooked	1 cup	15.6
Lima beans, cooked	1 cup	13.2
Peanuts	1 oz	2.3
Pistachio nuts	1 oz	3.1
Pumpkin seeds	¼ cup	4.1
Soybeans, cooked	1 cup	7.6
Sunflower seeds	¼ cup	3.0
Supplement: Metamucil	1 tsp	5.0

Adapted from commonsensehealth.com fiber rich foods

FATS

Not all fats are the same, nor do they have the same impact on inflammation in the body or on the joints. You may be familiar with saturated and unsaturated fats. Saturated fats are typically solid at room temperature (butter), and unsaturated fats are liquid at room temperature (olive oil). In general, you want to err toward eating unsaturated fats. When you are dining out, beware: If something is fried at a high temperature in corn, soy, canola, or sunflower oil, there is trouble within. All those polyunsaturated oils (PUFAs) become easily oxidized, or toxic, at increased temperatures—so avoid foods fried in PUFAs as much as possible. For the purpose of this book, it is enough to know that oxidized fats are those fats that injure the cells with which they come in contact (see Kanner 2007).

When cooking for yourself, monounsaturated fats, like a light olive oil (not extra-virgin), can withstand moderate heating, but when higher temperatures require a saturated oil, unrefined organic coconut oil is a good choice. It can give a slight coconut taste to fried food, but I think it is delicious!

It has been shown that specific unhealthy saturated fats are more inflammatory than specific healthy unsaturated fats. Improving your choice of specific fats and the ratio of saturated to unsaturated fats in your diet is an important step toward a joint-healthy life.

Trans fats (also known as trans-fatty acids) are found in many processed foods. Trans fats are derived from unsaturated oils heated at high temperatures. Trans fats are the result of processing vegetable oils and can be found in baked goods, chips, crackers, and deep-fried foods. They have a negative effect on "good" cholesterol, can lead to an increase in "bad" cholesterol, and are generally bad for your cardiovascular health. They cause inflammation and directly affect the inflammatory molecule TNF-alpha, which means they are not good for your joints, either. I encourage you to avoid trans-fatty acids like the plague, for your heart, for your joints, for your overall health! The secret key for detecting trans fats in a product is reading the ingredient label and looking for the code words *hydrogenated* – bad _____ oil. Soybean is the most common, but it can be any kind of unsaturated oil—vegetable, palm, or corn. If it says "hydrogenated _____ oil" on the label, drop the product like a hot rock! Trans fats act like sludge in the membranes, are inflammatory, and are joint unhealthy.

Once you know which fats to seek and which to avoid, you can take a closer look at which foods contain good and bad fats. The following chart will let you analyze the typical fat content of a range of foods.

UNSATURATED/SATURATED FAT CONTENT OF COMMON FOODS (100 grams = 3.5 ounces)			
Food		Unsaturated Fat (g)/100 g Food*	Saturated Fat (g)/100 g
MEAT			
Buffalo	(top round steak)	0.9	0.8
Beef	Ground (75 percent)		7.3
	Ground (85 percent)		5.9
	Rib		11.7
Lamb	Loin (¼" fat trim)	11.7	13
Pork	Bacon		13.7
	Rib		11.0
	Sausage		9.0
	Ham		6.0
	Chop		3.0
Chicken	Breast		1.0
	Dark meat		3.1
	Fried wing		5.8
Turkey	White	1.4	0.9
	Dark	2.3	1.5

UNSATURATED/SATURATED FAT CONTENT OF COMMON FOODS (100 grams = 3.5 ounces)		
Food	Unsaturated Fat (g)/100 g Food*	Saturated Fat (g)/100 g
FISH		
Salmon ✓	9.5	2.0
Halibut	1.9	0.4
Trout	1.8	0.7
Sardines	10.7	2.8
Snapper	0.9	0.4
Shrimp	0.9	0.3
Lobster	0.1	0.25
CHEESE		
American		19.7
Cream cheese		22.0
Cheddar		21.1
Swiss		17.8
Mozzarella (whole)		13.2
Mozzarella (skim)		12.7
Ricotta (whole)		8.3
Ricotta (skim)		4.9
Cottage		2.9
EGGS		
Eggs		2.6–4.0
Egg whites		0
DAIRY		
Butter ✓	24.0	51.4
VEGETABLE		
Olive oil ✓	83.5	13.8

* Foods with no value in the column have little to no unsaturated fats

From DietaryFiberFood.com; WeightLossForAll.com; www.nal.usda.gov/fnic/foodcomp/Data/

Here's something to think about: combining fats with carbohydrates slows down carbohydrate absorption. A small dollop of whipped cream with fresh berries, a little butter on a yam as a treat, or olive oil on broccoli makes what you're eating even healthier.

THE OMEGAS

No discussion of fats is complete without including the omegas. It is helpful to maximize omega-3 fat consumption while minimizing omega-6 fat consumption.

Omega-6 fats are found in animal products (meat, fish, dairy, and eggs), nuts, seeds, and vegetable oils. You also must be careful to minimize saturated fat consumption, while realizing that all saturated fats are not created equally.

- Myristic and palmitic fatty acids, more prevalent in grain-fed cattle, are much more detrimental than stearic fatty acid, which is more prevalent in grass-fed cattle. This is why it's better for your joints to eat grass-fed beef.
- In general, fish is better than land-animal meat. Eat wild salmon, not farm-raised salmon, to get the true omega-3s and the most beneficial ratio of saturated to unsaturated fats and vitamins. You want wild Alaskan sockeye salmon, if possible.
- Most cheeses, other than cottage cheese, aren't very good, although mozzarella and ricotta aren't so bad.
- Olive oil is a lot better than butter, and egg whites are fat free!

Just like the food that we eat affects our health, the food that animals eat affects their health in the same way. Salmon cannot produce omega-3s. They consume them in the plankton they eat. Farm-raised salmon and Atlantic salmon don't eat the same plankton that wild

Alaskan sockeye salmon eat. Therein lies the benefit of wild Alaskan sockeye salmon.

The same goes for grass-fed versus grain-fed cows. If you're going to eat beef, try to find beef from grass-fed cows. They provide a healthier fat profile. The saturated fats in grass-fed cows tend toward stearic fatty acid rather than myristic and palmitic fatty acids. It is quite simple: stearic acid is not as inflammatory as the other two fatty acids, and palmitic fatty acid, in particular, causes heightened cholesterol levels. If you are going to eat beef, remember that the steer to eat is the one with stearic acid—the grass-fed one. I highly recommend taking a look at Cynthia Daley's review of fatty acids, cited in the bibliography and available at www.healthyjointsforlife.com.

You have probably seen eggs on sale with the health claim "contains omega-3s" printed prominently on the carton. This claim is based on the fact that the chickens are fed a diet rich in omega-3s and thus produce eggs with omega-3s. The eggs with omega-3s are better for you, but they can be more expensive. If the cost seems prohibitive, you could eat regular eggs and take an omega-3 supplement. Do the math to see what works better for you.

PROTEINS

My advice is to eat protein liberally but also be conscious of the fats in meats. Meats are a high-protein food, which is great, but you may not want to eat 75 percent ground meat every night, because the saturated fat and the omega-6 unsaturated fat content that come with the protein in the ground meat are inflammatory. Watch for the sugar that can come with some protein sources. An eight-ounce serving of yogurt might give you five grams of good protein, but there may also be five grams of fat and thirty-four grams of inflammatory sugar in that eight-ounce serving. Always check the nutrition label to see what might accompany protein.

As you saw from the unsaturated/saturated fat chart, in general, fish is the best protein source, particularly salmon. Other preferred sources of protein are chicken, turkey, pork chops, and buffalo. As for other common meats, enjoy them sparingly. When you want beef, look for grass-fed beef for its improved saturated fat profile.

Other foods containing healthy amounts of protein also need to be evaluated carefully. For example, peanut butter has a good amount of protein, but some brands contain hydrogenated oils (i.e., trans fats), as well as lots of fat and a good amount of carbohydrates. I recommend that you eat "natural" peanut butter and avoid "regular" jarred peanut butter. Familiar brands of "natural" peanut butter are available in stores, so be sure to take a look. Always check the label. Trans fats are most definitely not "natural" and are specifically added to foods to enhance shelf life, so I think most people assume "natural" means no trans fats. Never assume. Even foods that say "trans fats = 0 g" can have .5 g.

The "Nutrition Facts" label tells you the amount of trans fats in the product. You need to know that the numbers are rounded off, and foods can contain fractional amounts of trans fats. For example, the label may show the quantity of trans fats as 0 grams, although the food really contains .45 grams. If the ingredients list includes a partially hydrogenated oil, don't eat the product. Small amounts of trans fats eaten multiple times over the course of a day can lead to several grams of trans fats in your daily diet—enough to sabotage your joint health. Reading labels can be tricky, because there is no standard definition of *natural* in the United States. Be sure to check the ingredients in a product to verify that you are getting what you need for joint health.

Eggs are another fantastic source of protein. However, the yolk contains substantial amounts of cholesterol and fat. I suggest eating

50 percent egg whites and 50 percent whole eggs to limit yolk consumption. But don't become crazed about skipping egg yolks, because nutrients, including many vitamins and choline, are highly concentrated in the yolk, and you don't want to miss out on these nutrients. Choline, also found in liver, cod, cruciferous vegetables, chicken, milk, soybeans, wheat germ, and tofu, plays a big role in cell membrane composition and is part of the molecules that are so important for nerve transmission.

Eating protein leads to a feeling of fullness (satiety) and slows carbohydrate absorption, so combining carbohydrates with proteins is preferred. Try broccoli and steak, chili with beans and ground meat, or sweet potato with chicken.

INSULIN

Any discussion about successfully managing carbohydrate digestion and metabolism must center on balancing insulin, the far-reaching hormonal hub of our system. Insulin is quite inflammatory and is secreted in direct response to blood sugar levels. If you want to avoid joint pain, blood sugar levels need to be minimized so insulin secretion is reduced and, therefore, inflammation is lessened. Less sugar means less insulin means less inflammation means less joint pain. Controlling glucose and insulin levels also helps prevent the stiffening of collagen, which is so damaging to our joints. Chronic increased insulin causes fluid retention, as well as weight gain, neither of which is beneficial to joints. In fact, fluid retention all by itself can make joints feel swollen and tight. Motion is restricted. Most of us know that feeling of a ring that is too tight after a night of "bad" eating, meaning consuming foods with lots of salt. Insulin isn't salt, but it causes that same type of fluid retention. We definitely need to avoid that.

It may be startling to learn how essential the hormone insulin is to the overall functioning of the human body. Its pervasiveness continually impresses me. In fact, its ubiquitous presence is the reason why the disease diabetes affects all organ systems. Insulin, produced in the beta cells of the pancreas, is secreted in response to blood sugar levels, which vary based on the absorption of sugar (glucose) into the bloodstream from foods we eat. Insulin controls the cell membrane channels that allow sugar to enter cells. The sugar glucose, as directed by insulin, comes out of the blood and into the cells, where it can be metabolized to create energy for cell use. Without insulin, the glucose cannot pass into the cells and be used for energy, growth, and other functions. Insulin's notoriety may come from its effect on sugar; however, it also impacts protein, fat, and cholesterol metabolism and balances the overall energy state of the body. Insulin is an incredibly important and powerful hormone.

Food that comes into the body is stored in cells as an energy source, namely, as glucose for immediate use; as glycogen in the liver for gradual, short-term use; and as fat everywhere for long-term storage. No surprise that sugar makes us fat! Insulin stimulates the production of fat-synthesizing enzymes as glucose levels rise. After all, if there is too much glucose available, then there needs to be a shift to longer-term storage. Once the fat-synthesizing enzymes are produced, the excess glucose is made into fat. Insulin also encourages the production of enzymes that store and create glycogen, which is the way glucose molecules are stored in the liver. Insulin has a central role in the production of the enzymes that make and break down fats and sugar. We can help control insulin levels by controlling the amount and types of carbohydrates that we eat.

The effects of insulin on human liver cells show that insulin alone, without glucose, causes inflammation. While insulin and glucose are intimately related in the body, one specific part of a classic study by M. Okazaki isolated insulin from glucose to investigate the effect of insulin alone on inflammation. All by itself insulin increased inflammation. People who become insensitive to insulin (usually from obesity) and therefore need the additional secretion of insulin to control blood sugar levels are necessarily living with excessive inflammation.

Imagine walking into your grandparents' house to find the TV blaring. Grandma and Grandpa are ten feet in front of the TV, completely unaware of the deafening volume. Grandma and Grandpa don't hear well, so they simply turn up the volume. The same thing happens to cells as they become less sensitive to insulin. Cells get to a point where they don't "hear" normal amounts of insulin. To satisfy the cells, the pancreas simply secretes more insulin and thereby bathes the cells in an excess of insulin. Just like Grandma and Grandpa can hear the TV only at deafening volumes, the cells absorb glucose only when bathed in egregious amounts of insulin. The problem is that there is more inflammation provoking Insulin circulating as cells become less sensitive to insulin.

This is what happens with diabetes: either less insulin is secreted by the pancreas because the pancreas isn't working well or the individual cells become resistant to insulin, necessitating more insulin from the pancreas. As cells become resistant, the cell glucose channels (especially muscle cells, which absorb so much glucose) don't open up as easily, so glucose can't get into the cells. Even more specifically, it is the actual cell receptors located on the cell membrane that change shape, so when insulin tries to connect to the receptors, the lock and key mechanisms don't work. This is insulin resistance.

GOOD ADVICE

When I was a third-year medical student, some of my rotations were at the VA hospital in West Haven, Connecticut, a Yale-affiliated hospital where I would also rotate during my orthopedic residency. My first rotation was in

continued

internal medicine, under attending physician Rosemary Fisher. With the tenderness of a mother and the brilliance of a sage, Dr. Fisher made me understand what a privilege it is to treat patients. I was reserved and nervous when I first started, so Dr. Fisher gave me some advice that was simple, but that I have never forgotten. She reinforced the idea that our job was serious, but she also stressed that it was okay to smile and enjoy helping patients. The intern she assigned to watch over me was an amazing, poised young doctor named Silvio Inzucchi. Dr. Inzucchi was extremely bright and exceptionally patient with all the students, especially me. I quietly looked at him and said to myself, *That's the kind of doctor I want to be.* Silvio wrote a chapter on diabetes in 2011 (which I cite in the bibliography) that is a quintessential reference and tells you all about insulin resistance.

In the above-mentioned Okazaki study, researchers tried to understand what was happening in the body in real-life situations when insulin is mixed with inflammatory messengers. Interleukin-1 beta, tumor necrosis factor, and matrix metalloproteinases (MMPs) are some of our inflammatory foes. When insulin was added to liver cells bathed in pro-inflammatory interleukin-1 beta (an inflammatory messenger), the production of inflammatory molecules was substantially magnified. Remember that MMPs are particularly cartilage destructive—they are akin to battery acid for joints. This study clearly established that high levels of insulin put the body in an inflammatory state, which is clearly undesirable for decreasing joint pain.

Iwasaki's 2007 study reported in the *Journal of Diabetes Complications* showed that high glucose levels in the presence of insulin caused a 40 percent increase in NFkB activity. Insulin alone is inflammatory, glucose alone is inflammatory, and when they are together in the body, they operate synergistically to create problems. Clearly, insulin and glucose are pro-inflammatory culprits that need to be controlled and apprehended before they rob us of our joint health.

INSULIN AND CARBOHYDRATES

Foods like bread, pasta, beans, potatoes, rice, vegetables, and fruits are examples of carbohydrates. They are digested in our gastrointestinal tract and break down into the simple sugars: fructose, galactose, and glucose. Whether you eat a banana, lettuce, or a candy bar, only fructose, galactose, and glucose are produced.

Glucose is the sugar reported to us in blood tests. It is absorbed into the bloodstream and delivered to the body as an energy source. Insulin is necessary to maintain blood sugar levels, which it does by allowing sugar to enter cells through channels or pores in the cell membrane. Without insulin, blood sugar levels rise and the disease process of diabetes occurs. Diabetes is a particularly onerous disease because of the effect sugar has on tissues—see page 34, AGEs.

Fructose is often used as a commercial sweetener, because it is two and a half times as sweet as glucose. It is also the sugar with the worst reputation. During digestion, it is not as well absorbed as glucose and will ferment in the large intestine, causing gas and bloating. Certainly not the best thing for a cocktail party! Other sugars don't cause the same extent of bloating or gas. Fructose also increases triglyceride levels, because it is metabolized to dihydroxyacetone phosphate (DHAP), which is then used to produce triglyceride fats, prime perpetrators of heart disease. People who consume fructose have higher triglyceride blood levels than those on diets predominated by glucose or simple sugars. Interestingly, fructose does not cause insulin secretion like glucose. Glucose has the lock-and-key shape to attach to pancreas cells and cause these cells to make and secrete insulin; fructose does not have that shape. Fructose does, however, have a huge impact on proteins. It can attach itself to proteins ten to fifteen times more readily than glucose. Fructose's ability to attach to proteins, like collagen or elastin, results in damage to cells and tissues that contain those important proteins, such as tendons and ligaments. Kids need to stay away from soda and drinks with high fructose sugar (usually called high fructose corn syrup, or HFCS) for three very good reasons:

1 It makes them fat.
2 It increases their blood triglyceride levels.
3 It attacks their joint collagen and elastin.

HFCS impacts joints negatively over time because of its effect on collagen. Fructose is a carb and is bad for the reasons cited above, even though it doesn't increase insulin levels. Table sugar is called sucrose and is made of glucose and fructose. Table sugar has both glucose and fructose in a 1:1 ratio. Table sugar, therefore, can deliver all the bad effects of glucose, as well as those of fructose.

Glucose actually has the ability to bond two substances together. If there are high glucose levels in your system, the glucose will bond adjacent collagen molecules, preventing them from engaging in normal fluid motion. Advanced glycation end products (AGEs) are an indication of the "aging" effect of glucose on tissues made of collagen, like ligaments, cartilage, and skin. Just like a child gets sticky fingers from the sugar in cotton candy, glycated collagen is stiff and sticky. Glucose damages collagen in joint ligaments and/ or causes cartilage to become glycated and stiff. An "aging" joint is an excellent example of a glycated, stiff joint. I'm sure you have seen the leathery appearance of skin when it loses its elasticity. It sags, wrinkles, and shows signs of aging. Now imagine that the very same thing that is happening to skin is happening to joint ligaments and cartilage.

It is so important to try to keep sugar levels moderate to prevent the damaging effects that too much sugar has on your system. But remember, too little sugar and a person can faint from hypoglycemia (low blood glucose levels). Too much sugar and the glycation of collagen and other tissues occurs, along with an increased risk for diabetes.

WHAT A BLIND MAN HEARD— THE EFFECTS OF DIABETES

During my orthopedic residency, while at the same VA hospital in West Haven, Connecticut, where years before I had met the great Drs. Rosemary Fisher and Silvio Inzucchi, I had the opportunity to meet countless veterans who had given so much to our country. Many of them suffered from the physical torments of war. It was our job to help them. Moreover, it was our privilege.

Every day my patient Mr. Camp and I had a standing meeting. I'd walk into his room exactly at 5:45 a.m. to draw blood and perform an arterial blood gas. The ward was usually quiet at this early hour. Mr. Camp was a veteran of World War II and had developed terrible diabetes, which led to circulatory problems, as well as arthritis, heart disease, kidney disease, and blindness. Mr. Camp never knew what I looked like, but he knew me each morning by the sound of my sneakers. He could pick up the faint squeak of the rubber on the VA hospital's polished tiles. Sometimes I'd walk in with a nurse, and Mr. Camp would ask, "Who'd you bring with you today, Dr. Diana?" Inevitably, each morning I'd walk into his room and he'd greet me with an optimistic, "Good morning, Dr. Diana. I hope your aim is good today."

Patients with diabetes sometimes are particularly difficult blood draws. Mr. Camp was a vasculopath, which meant that his vessels were in really bad shape. Drawing blood from him was a nightmare. Getting the blood from his veins was tough, but I used special techniques to minimize his pain. Mr. Camp appreciated my special techniques and enjoyed our daily talks. He also had a great sense of humor. One day he asked me if I knew why he liked me so much, and before I could muster an answer, he said, "Don't get carried away. Mostly, it's because you usually hit on the first needle stick." More than once Mr. Camp begged me, "Please be my William Tell."

Mr. Camp's diabetes could not be cured. His disease was far enough along so that its far-reaching effects couldn't be reversed, either. Fortunately, we helped him enough to get him out of the VA hospital and back to his home. He appreciated that more than most might imagine. On his day of discharge he told me something I'll never forget. "You're a good man, Richard Diana. You helped me with patience and skill. I'll never forget the sound of your gentle, caring footsteps." Like I said, taking care of patients is a privilege.

THE GLYCEMIC INDEX AND GLYCEMIC LOAD

The glycemic index (GI) and glycemic load (GL) help us to understand how specific carbohydrates influence blood sugar levels and in turn impact insulin levels. These concepts helps in choosing which carbohydrates are joint healthy.

The GI is a measure of a carbohydrate's ability, when consumed, to make blood glucose levels rise. In the GI all foods are measured relative to glucose and its impact on blood sugar. Glucose has a rating of one hundred on the glycemic index. The higher the glycemic index of a food, the higher the glucose spike will be when it is digested. I recommend that you try to eat foods with a lower GI to prevent glucose spikes. However, there are variables you should consider beyond the GI rating. For example, eating twice as much of a food with a GI of fifty is equivalent to having consumed a food with a GI of one hundred. The ripeness of a food (think brown versus green bananas) and the consistency of a food (think mashed potatoes versus whole potatoes) affect the GI, as well. The riper and more mashed up a food is, the higher its GI tends to be.

While the glycemic index is quite useful, the glycemic load is a better predictor of the effect of a food on blood sugar and insulin, because the GL also factors in the number of grams of carbohydrates in the food (carbohydrate density). Thus the key difference between the GI and the GL is that the glycemic load takes into account the portion size and the food's glycemic index. For example, it is unlikely that a person would eat a large bowl of corn, but it is common for a person to eat a large bowl of whole-grain pasta. Although the pasta has a lower glycemic index than corn, because we tend to eat it in larger quantities, the pasta has a greater effect on blood sugar levels. So, pasta is better than corn, but only if you watch your portions. It's a slight oversimplification, but basically, to calculate the GL of a carbohydrate, multiply the GI by the number of grams.

How a food is prepared can also impact the GI and the GL. Foods that take longer to digest cause less of a glucose spike than those that are more quickly digested, and so they are preferable. A whole potato is better than a whole mashed potato. Instant mashed potatoes are the worst, because they are so finely ground. Their increased surface area makes it easier for the intestine to absorb them quickly.

More thoroughly cooked foods usually have a higher GI. When eating pasta, consider the lower GI of al dente (firm) pasta versus the higher GI of softer, overboiled pasta. Also, consider the lower GI of thicker linguini compared to thinner angel-hair pasta. The smaller the pieces, the more easily they are digested.

It is important to realize that combining carbohydrates with either fats or proteins slows down absorption and thereby reduces the GI. By reducing the GI, you are effectively curbing the amount of inflammation-provoking insulin in your system. Joints feel better without inflammation.

Various food groups are discussed below from the vantage point of their GI ratings. Each is followed by a list of foods and their GI. The lower the number, the better. I have included these foods because they are joint healthy by virtue of their low GI and they are popular foods that you should have no trouble buying at your local supermarket. They will be excellent choices for the eight-week program.

Fruits

If you choose fruits with a GI of less than fifty, you will have a delicious list of choices. The fruits that are less than fifty on the GI scale, which include berries, are full of incredible antioxidants. Remember portion size and density count. A whole banana might weigh twice as much as a bunch of strawberries of equal volume. It's best to eat fresh fruits, so stay away from calorie-dense dried fruits. Although they haven't been formally tested, I don't hesitate in recommending berries, such as blueberries, raspberries, and blackberries. It's estimated that they have a GI of forty, similar to strawberries. If you pair berries with a dollop of whipped cream or plain yogurt, their GI rating will decrease, as the topping slows the berries' absorption.

GLYCEMIC INDEX FOR 50 G PORTION	
Cherries	22
Grapefruit	25
Prunes	29
Apricots	30
Apples	38
Peaches (canned in juice)	38
Pears (fresh)	38
Plums	39
Strawberries	40
Oranges	42
Peaches (fresh)	42
Grapes	46
Mangos	51

Bananas	52
Papaya	56
Raisins	56
Apricots	57
Kiwis	58
Figs (dried)	61
Cantaloupe	65
Pineapple (fresh)	66
Watermelon	72
Dates	103

Vegetables

It is amazing how many vegetables have a GI of only ten! They are an incredibly versatile group and can be used in salads and as sides and toppings. How about lettuce, onions, and sautéed mushrooms on top of a buffalo burger? How about a salad with a mix of shredded cabbage, romaine lettuce, and red peppers, topped with some rosemary-infused olive oil? Vegetables also have lots of fiber, which we absolutely *love!*

GLYCEMIC INDEX FOR 50 G PORTION	
Broccoli	10
Cabbage	10
Lettuce	10
Mushrooms	10
Onions	10
Red peppers	10
Green peas	48
Carrots	49
Corn	60
Beets	64

continued

GLYCEMIC INDEX FOR 50 G PORTION	
Pumpkin	75
Parsnips	97

Potatoes

Yams and sweet potatoes have wonderfully low GIs! Knowing the GIs of potatoes, which vary according to how they are prepared, makes choosing a healthy potato dish easy. If you succumb to the temptation of mashed potatoes, please stay away from the instant variety. Your joints will thank you. At dinner one night at the home of friends, they substituted baked breaded parsnips for French fried potatoes because they knew I am careful about what I eat. The parsnips were delicious, and because they weren't fried, they seemed to be a better choice than the French fries. But when I got home and checked the GI of parsnips, I was shocked! Don't be fooled into eating too many parsnips, which have a GI of ninety-seven, even if they are offered in place of French fries. Baked, not fried, sweet potato fries are a better substitute.

GLYCEMIC INDEX FOR 50 G PORTION	
Yams	37
Sweet potatoes	44
French fries	75
Baked (white potato)	85
Instant mashed	86
Boiled (red skin)	88

Pasta

The GIs of pastas are fairly low, but remember what we said previously about the glycemic load. We tend to eat a sizable amount of pasta, so beware of the portion size. Remember that the GI is based on fifty grams of carbs, so read your labels carefully. Also, you should give low-carbohydrate pastas a try. We've used low-carb pasta at my house for years, and none of my Italian relatives have ever protested!

GLYCEMIC INDEX FOR 50 G PORTION	
Egg fettuccine	32
Whole wheat spaghetti	37
White spaghetti	38
Linguini	46
Capellini	47
Macaroni	47
Rice vermicelli	58

Breads

You may be surprised to see that some 100 percent whole wheat breads have a GI the same or even higher than white bread. Any grain, including wheat, that is ground into flour will have a GI similar to white bread. Many wheat breads also contain molasses for coloring and taste. Since molasses is a by-product of heating sugar its presence increases GI even further. Bread made from whole wheat that is minimally ground will have larger particles that are more difficult to digest so it will have a lower GI. If the first ingredient on the bread label is (any grain) *flour,* then the bread's GI will be high. If the first ingredient is *ground whole wheat,* instead of whole wheat flour, it will be better.

Not appearing on this list are sprouted breads, like Ezekiel 4:9, which have not been tested but are likely superior to breads made with flour. If we know that sprouts have a good GI and that there isn't a lot of flour in a specific bread, then we know the GI of that bread will be better. However, sprouted breads are dense, so beware of their glycemic load. A half-inch slice may weigh 50 percent more than flour-based bread. The GI of sprouted bread may be 30 percent better than a different bread, but the amount usually eaten may be 50 percent more, hence the sprouted bread that you thought was better for you ends up increasing your blood sugar. The numbers may be a little confusing at first, but it's actually simple once you get the hang of it.

GLYCEMIC INDEX FOR 50 G PORTION	
Pumpernickel	41
Ground whole wheat	53
Hamburger bun	61
Croissant	67
White	70
Bagel	72
Whole wheat 100%	77
French baguette	95

Baked Goods

Because of the high GI of many baked goods, if you are going to eat them, it is best if you can make your own treats using lower glycemic ground hulled flours found in natural food stores. Look for coarsely ground or stone ground, but not finely ground, flour. Mesquite pods, from the Southwest, might be interesting to experiment with. They can be found in natural food stores and on the internet (for example, Dowd & Rogers mesquite pod flour), or they can be purchased directly from Arizona producers, such as Skeleton Creek/The Mesquitery in Aravaipa Canyon, Arizona, and Bean Tree Farm in Tucson, Arizona.

Many products and packaged goods are labeled "gluten free" (gluten is a protein in wheat and other grains), but they can contain corn, potato, rice, and other high GI ingredients. Almond flour is a good example of an exotic flour that has a lower GI. It is great in baked goods, especially macaroons! Remember that a high GI is a result of the way a grain is ground as much as the actual grain itself. The numbers below for baked goods made with typical flour, could be radically different if a different, less finely ground flour were used. Buy some mesquite pods or use some almond flour and experiment.

GLYCEMIC INDEX FOR 50 G PORTION	
Blueberry muffin	59
Bran muffin	60
Carrot muffin	62
Doughnut	76
Scone	92

From www.lowglycemicdiet.com

Dairy Products

The low GI of ice cream is an excellent example of how fat slows down the absorption of carbohydrates and leads to a lower GI. Yogurt is great for smoothies when blended with berries, protein powder, and ice.

GLYCEMIC INDEX FOR 50 G PORTION	
Yogurt (artificially sweetened with stevia)	14
Whole milk	31
Skim milk	32
Sugar-sweetened yogurt	33
Ice cream	38
Low-fat ice cream	43

Beans

Beans are high in complex carbohydrates and dietary fiber. Dried chickpeas can be ground into flour, while fresh chickpeas are the foundation for hummus. Sliced cucumbers and hummus are a wonderful alternative to chips and dips. Lentils can add protein and fiber to soups. I like to add kidney beans to buffalo chili for flavor and added fiber.

GLYCEMIC INDEX FOR 50 G PORTION	
Chickpeas (dried)	28
Lentils	29
Lima beans	32
Chickpeas (canned)	42
Baked beans	48
Kidney beans (canned)	52

Rice and Grains

Barley is a great addition to soup, especially with chicken breast. Hulled barley, in which only the outer hull is removed, is better than pearled barley where processing removes the bran. Hulled barley is fiber rich and has a high concentration of tocotrienols, an especially joint-healthy form of vitamin E. In general, rice should not be considered joint healthy.

GLYCEMIC INDEX FOR 50 G PORTION	
Pearled barley	25
Converted white rice	38
Long-grain white rice	44
Hulled barley	50
Buckwheat	54

Brown rice	55
Couscous	65
Cornmeal	68
Short-grain white rice	72
Instant white rice	87
Wild rice	87
Sticky rice (white)	98

Beverages

Hydration is important for joint health. Water should be your go-to beverage, while high-calorie sodas, energy drinks, and sports drinks should be avoided. Drink water regularly, at least seventy-two ounces per day. In the eight-week plan section we deal with this more specifically. Try to avoid drinking artificially sweetened drinks, like diet sodas and waters enhanced with vitamins. Don't waste your money trying to get your vitamins from flavored waters. There are less costly and better ways to get vitamins. There are questions about the effect of diet sodas on insulin secretion. If you want to drink a carbonated beverage, drink seltzer.

I don't believe in drinking coffee, because it is addicting. There is no specific data suggesting it is unhealthy for joints, but seeing its addicting effects on surgical patients who are forced to fast overnight has led me to be a big opponent of coffee. Coffee drinkers, after simply skipping their morning coffee, will have headaches, nausea, and mental stress. Anything that causes such incapacity should be avoided. If you've been drinking coffee for years, try to reduce your coffee consumption, if not for joint health, then just to rid yourself of an unnecessary addictive behavior.

On the other hand, I've never seen tea drinkers have similar symptoms, although tea also has caffeine, albeit in smaller quantities. Substituting tea for coffee might be a viable option for some. Green tea is a healthy drink that should be consumed daily for its antioxidant benefits and its effects on metabolism (i.e., speeding it up). In addition, important studies indicate that green tea suppresses NFkB and twenty-nine inflammatory proteins that NFkB produces.

Juices

Note that juices, with the exception of pineapple juice, have a higher GI than their respective whole fruits. While a glass of fresh juice can be delicious, the whole fruit is preferred for joint health, because of the fiber content of the whole fruit. The lower GI translates into less inflammation-provoking insulin in your system.

GLYCEMIC INDEX FOR 50 G PORTION	
Tomato	38
Apple	40
Pineapple	46
Grapefruit	48
Orange	53
Cranberry	68

Sweeteners

Regular sugar sweeteners should not be consumed in any quantity if you want to control insulin levels. I suggest using a sweetener made from the stevia plant as a sugar substitute. It can be added to coffee (but try to kick the habit!), tea, and other beverages, and you can cook with it. Sweeteners like sucralose and aspartame (both with a GI of zero) may cause some insulin secretion, so I recommend avoiding them. I use Truvia almost exclusively, but some people complain of a bitter aftertaste. That deserves some explanation: Stevia-based sweeteners are made of rebaudioside and stevioside. Stevioside is bitter tasting, and so the stevia sweetener you select should have more rebaudioside and less stevioside (check the label). The Truvia brand also has erythritol in it, which is a sugar alcohol, but, as you will learn in the section below on sugar alcohols, doesn't cause diarrhea. Erythritol has a cool taste on the tongue. Truvia, with more rebaudioside and some erythritol, may be as appealing to you as it is to me. I sprinkle it on whole grapefruit for breakfast. Delicious.

Agave nectar is also a popular sugar substitute. It is made from the same agave plant used to make tequila, and is primarily produced in Mexico. Unfortunately, there can be variability in production methods and quality control. Many consider agave nectar natural and raw, but this may not be the case, because it is heated beyond 118°F to mature the sugars. Agave is predominantly fructose, which we know is joint unhealthy because of its ability to glycate collagen (AGEs). It is also heart unhealthy because it forms the backbone for triglycerides.

A study conducted in 2010 on mice, not humans, by Nemoseck showed that agave was a better alternative than sucrose (table sugar) when it came to weight gain and insulin sensitivity. That certainly should be considered, but we are desperately trying to avoid sucrose, so the fact that agave is better is only a mild compliment. The GI of agave nectar is deceptively low but certainly not as low as stevia. I believe we should be skeptical of agave as a joint-healthy alternative to sugar. Therefore, I prefer stevia over other sweeteners because of its effect not only on joints, but also on overall health.

GLYCEMIC INDEX FOR 50 G PORTION	
Stevia (Truvia)	0
Lactose	19
Agave nectar	30
Maple syrup	54
Honey	55
Table sugar (sucrose)	67

continued

GLYCEMIC INDEX FOR 50 G PORTION	
Pancake syrup	76
Glucose	100

Sugar Alcohols

One of the great failures of "low-carbohydrate" diets is their inability to satisfy sugar cravings. Virtually everyone wants an occasional piece of candy or chocolate cake. Sugar alcohols can be a saving grace for those times, so this discussion of sugar alcohols could be quintessential for the success of this joint relief program. Sugar alcohols are aptly named because they are sweet. The following chart depicts the relative sweetness of various sugars and sugar alcohols. Note that if it ends in -*ose*, it's a sugar, and if it ends in -*ol*, it's a sugar alcohol.

SUGAR ALCOHOLS' SWEETNESS COMPARED TO TABLE SUGAR'S SWEETNESS	
Relative sweetness*	
Sucrose (table sugar)	100
Xylitol	100
Maltitol	90
Erythritol	81
Glucose	74
Sorbitol	55
Isomalt	50

* This scale indicates that isomalt, at 50, is half as sweet as sucrose, at 100.

Adapted from scientificpsychic.com

All of the above sugar alcohols are found in sugar-free foods, including candy. The reason we are interested in sugar alcohols is that they are sweet, don't cause insulin secretion, and are almost 50 percent lower in calories than sugars. The additional good news is that they have received certification from the FDA as "generally recognized as safe" (GRAS). The biggest problem with sugar alcohols is that they (with the exception of erythritol) are not absorbed in the small intestine and are passed on to the large intestine, where they cause large intestine lining cells to secrete water, leading to diarrhea. It turns out that 90 percent of erythritol is absorbed by the small intestine and thus does not cause gastrointestinal upset, except in large quantities. Sugar alcohols may be helpful for your sweet tooth, but one must be careful of the gastrointestinal effects! Erythritol is better tolerated than maltitol, sorbitol, and xylitol, and it is almost as sweet as regular sugar (see Oku 2002 for more specific information on sugar alcohols). In addition, intestinal bacteria digest sugar alcohols into short-chain fatty acids. Thus they start out with the name "sugar" but end up via digestion as fat, courtesy of the bacteria that live in your intestines. The caloric content of sugar alcohols, which is 50 percent less than a sugar, therefore comes from the short-chain fats that they become.

INSULIN AND FATS

Insulin promotes the storage of the sugar, glucose, in the liver so that it can later be released to the body to use as fuel. Glucose is stored in the liver as glycogen for gradual and short-term use. For long-term storage, glucose is converted to fat.

When the liver is saturated with glycogen, excess glucose is transformed into fatty acids by an enzyme called fatty acid synthase (FAS). The liver combines the fat ("lipo" in medical talk) that is formed with carrier proteins, and these lipoproteins are exported into the blood. This process explains how too much sugar ingestion leads to fat in the blood (as well as on your backside), something you definitely want to avoid! This also explains what happens when people following a low-fat diet and indiscriminately consuming too many carbohydrates have blood tests that show increased fat levels (triglycerides). They don't understand how the blood test results could indicate worsening triglycerides (fat) or how their weight could be increasing. The cause is excess carbohydrates being converted to fat by FAS.

Insulin is intimately associated with producing fat and controlling the body's energy state. Fat metabolism is specifically controlled in the cell by insulin's effect on a DNA caretaker called sterol regulatory element-binding protein (SREBP). SREBP is an inactive membrane-bound protein waiting for activation by insulin or other stimuli. When it is activated, it goes to the nucleus and binds the DNA genes that produce enzymes necessary for making lipids, including FAS. A lifestyle of constant carbohydrate consumption causes persistent elevated insulin levels. This signals the cell to make FAS and other lipid-creating enzymes. Eat too many carbohydrates and those excess carbs are made into fat via the SREBP-directed fat-synthesizing enzymes. This molecular pathway helps to explain why we can get fat by eating carbohydrates. Remember, gaining weight puts more pressure on your joints, and if you have arthritis, your cushioning is lessened. More pressure on less cushion means pain! Now you can amaze your friends with your metabolic knowledge and quiz your doctor next time you see him or her. Molecular knowledge is contagious!

INSULIN AND CHOLESTEROL

Three-quarters of the cholesterol in your blood is made by your body. Only one-quarter is a result of the food you eat. If you consume absolutely no cholesterol, the body will sense the lower cholesterol level and will activate cholesterol synthesis.

If you eat low-cholesterol and low-fat foods—meaning you eat more carbohydrates—you will stimulate more insulin production, which in turn generates a protein (SREBP) and an enzyme (HMG-CoA reductase) that cause cholesterol synthesis. Ironically, low-fat diets can cause your cholesterol levels—and the size of your love handles—to increase. If you intentionally avoid eating all foods that contain cholesterol, you would expect your cholesterol level to drop precipitously. Unfortunately, SREBP doesn't allow that to happen, because it stimulates your body to make more cholesterol. In terms of joint health, insulin leads to fat production, and extra weight overloads joints. Fat (lipoproteins) also clogs arteries via cholesterol production (especially bad cholesterol), therefore leading to the poor delivery of blood and oxygen throughout the body. Without optimum blood circulation and oxygen delivery, your ability to move is inhibited. Research has shown that insulin all by itself, and especially with high glucose levels, increases NFkB activity. This information further reinforces how joint unhealthy high levels of insulin can be, and why we need to control carbohydrate consumption.

INSULIN AND PROTEINS

It has been known for almost a century that insulin causes the cells to draw in amino acids and that these amino acids are the building blocks for proteins.

Insulin helps get amino acids into our cells, where they can help the cell run efficiently. Bodybuilders use this concept to great advantage. Before lifting, they will drink a fast-absorbing amino acid drink, along with a high GI sugar, like a soda, fruit drink, or energy drink. The sugar causes an insulin spike, and the high insulin levels open up muscle cell membranes for amino acid uptake. Amino acids are then available as building blocks for muscle growth.

THE YANKEES, THE METS, THE RED SOX, TED, AND ME

I grew up in a Yankee household. My father loved Joe DiMaggio more than life itself, while my brother, Vinny, was a devoted Mickey Mantle disciple. At the time, circa the 1960s, there were only six identifiable stations on our TV set. I guess our antenna wasn't the best. The Yanks were on WPIX, Channel 11, which had a weak signal, but it was good enough to watch the games. In my younger days, the Yanks were brutally bad, but I loved them just the same. I didn't know enough about the game to recognize that Horace Clark, Jerry Kenny, and Stick Michaels weren't the best ballplayers. They were Yankees. Dad and Mom told me countless stories about their World Series days with Yogi and Rizzuto, Ford and Martin and, of course, Joe D. My dad made sure that I knew that there would never be another ballplayer like Joe D. My folks, Vinny, and my sister, Marilyn, all loved (well, not so much my sister) the Yanks, and so I did too.

On many occasions my bedtime came before the game was over, so my brother, Vinny, almost eleven years my senior, would send me messages with the score. Our house was small and was designed so that my bedroom and my bed were only one thin wall and five feet away from the TV. My mother, father, and brother watched the game literally only ten feet away from where I was "sleeping." Vinny would sneak over to my bedroom door and softly announce the score. I knew my parents were close by, but I thought they didn't realize what Vinny and I were doing. I thought we were getting away with grand larceny. It made the games all the more sweet. It wasn't until thirty years later that I would learn the truth, that my mom and dad knew what was going on all along.

I was a tried-and-true Yankee fan until 1983. That all ended when my best friend from Yale, Ron Darling, started playing with the NY Mets. I certainly loved the Yanks, but Ronnie was blood, and as the saying goes, blood is thicker than water. I was a devoted Mets fan all through medical school, listening on my clock radio to Mets games while I studied in my twelve-foot-by-fourteen-foot luxury dorm room, complete with bed, desk, and illegal toaster oven. I saw Bill Buckner blow the ground ball at first base in the sixth game of the 1986 World Series while I was taking "call" as a sub-intern at Yale–New Haven Hospital. Since I had given Ronnie tickets for "my Super Bowl," Ronnie came through with tickets for me for "his World Series." The group of four young doctors sitting on cots in the on-call room screamed when the Mets won Game Six, forcing a deciding Game Seven, which Ronnie would start. And just days later all of us were there watching Ronnie and the Mets beat the Boston Red Sox to win the World Series.

My allegiance to the Mets never fully faded, but it was significantly weakened when, in my senior year of medical school, only months after the World Series, I met Dr. Arthur Pappas, minority owner and team physician of the Boston Red Sox. Dr. Pappas took me under his wing and over the next several years adopted me as a part of the Red Sox organization. I worked as a team orthopedic consultant from 1992 to 1998. If you follow my lineage, I started as a Yankee fan, changed to the Mets with Ronnie and rooted against the Red Sox in the '86 World Series, and just a few short years later became an actual part of the Red Sox organization. What a wild ride. Not bad for a former NFL player!

During one spring training, when I was a part of the Red Sox medical staff, I was approaching the clubhouse door when it suddenly swung open, nearly knocking me over. The older gentleman opening the door couldn't have been more apologetic. He was a big guy, standing at least half a foot above my five-foot-ten-inch frame, a porkpie hat on his head filled with flies for fly-fishing. He called me "Doc," so I figured he knew me. I was stunned when he grabbed me by the shoulders with the grip of a defensive lineman and asked if I was okay. I joked with him, saying that I'd been hit harder and that I was fine. I walked into the clubhouse, and five feet inside was Dr. Pappas, who had been watching the whole thing. He said to me, "I see you just met Ted." I looked at him bewildered, so he added, "Ted, Ted Williams. You've heard of him, haven't you?"

MY FAVORITE JOINT-HEALTHY FOODS

An analysis of the saturated and unsaturated fat content of various protein sources reveals that in order to stay joint healthy, you should eat proteins like salmon, chicken, turkey, pork chops, and buffalo. Carbohydrates and insulin can be inflammatory and should form a limited part of your diet. The GI and the GL may be confusing at first, but I'm sure in time you will become comfortable with this important approach to evaluating foods. There are many delicious joint-healthy vegetables that are high in fiber and phytonutrients (plant-based nutrients) and that won't spike your blood glucose.

I'm going to introduce you to some of my favorite extremely joint-healthy foods and drinks, which you shouldn't miss. Whether you cook or not, here are some of my favorite foods that are not only tasty but will also be beneficial to your joints—as well as your overall health. Think of these when you are planning your next meal.

CHICKEN'S BEST FRIEND: URSOLIC ACID

I love when my wife makes roasted chicken with rosemary and thyme. She meticulously rubs a mixture of olive oil, rosemary, and thyme under the skin of the chicken. Chicken is a wonderful source of lean protein, olive oil is a healthy monounsaturated oil, and the thyme offers subtle but distinct flavor. The chicken is mouthwatering, and I can't help but love it all the more, knowing how joint healthy it is. The best part, though, is the rosemary, which not only smells so delicious but also provides incredible joint health benefits. Rosemary comes from a plant that is teeming with ursolic acid and its close relative oleanolic acid. Both of these components of rosemary have been used over the centuries in Asian folk medicine for their antimicrobial, antiviral, and liver protection. Animal studies have shown they reduce inflammation in several different ways. Studies done in 2003 (Shishodia), 2006 (Lee), 2007 (Pathak), and 2012 (Checker) reveal that ursolic acid, if ingested, has the ability to inhibit NFkB, the linchpin of inflammation, and it specifically inhibits Nfat, another inflammatory DNA caretaker. In these studies ursolic acid was able to decrease the number of those nasty cytokines that play a pivotal role in breaking down the very stuff cartilage is made of.

ITALIAN TOMATO SAUCE AND GARLIC, AKA "THE SAUCE"

In my joint-healthy household, tomato sauce is started early in the morning, after church, with garlic simmering in olive oil, followed by chicken sausage, pork chops, grass-fed beef ribs, and buffalo meatballs. The crushed tomatoes and seasonings simmer with the lightly browned meats in a giant pot for hours. Sometimes there is a price to be paid for eating a bowl of pasta covered with a fantastic garlic-based tomato sauce. For some who typically eat more than their fair share, the garlic causes stomach upset, or "agita," as Tony Soprano or my grandpa Bellucci might call it. Despite the indigestion, many of my overzealous relatives are willing to pay the price for the taste of the homemade sauce.

I'm happy that the garlic in the sauce has never bothered me, because allicin, the active component in garlic, has been shown to suppress NFkB, TNF-alpha, and iNOS (the enzyme that leads to nitric oxide production) (see Hasan 2007). It also appears to be able to prevent T-cell (a type of white blood cell) adhesions to blood vessel walls, so it is heart-healthy and anti-inflammatory. Garlic should definitely be part of a joint-healthy anti-inflammatory diet. You can try garlic in supplement form, as well, but many of my patients (me too) complain of stomach upset, so be warned.

Don't forget that you don't want to eat your joint-healthy sauce with standard high-glycemic pasta. Select thicker varieties of pasta (e.g., fettuccine instead of angel-hair pasta), and cook it so that it is al dente. Over the years low-carb pasta has tricked every one of my relatives and friends (some of whom were born in Italy) who have eaten at my house. Don't think for a moment that low-carb pasta doesn't taste good.

ASTAXANTHIN AND SALMON

Salmon can be prepared in many ways. I like to cook it on the grill, in a tinfoil vessel, with a topping of capers and diced tomatoes. If it's easier for you, try this dish in the oven. Simply place the salmon on the tinfoil and garnish with capers and diced tomatoes. Fold the tinfoil to enclose the salmon, forming a little house, and leave it on the grill or in the oven for about ten minutes. You will have a delicious, moist, and tender protein source that is rich in omega-3s and astaxanthin, an incredible phytonutrient that gives salmon its orange/red color and is one hundred times as potent as vitamin E.

CRUCIFEROUS VEGETABLES

Broccoli and cauliflower are probably the most famous cruciferous vegetables, but cabbage lovers might challenge me on that one. Bok choy, collard greens, kale, horseradish, wasabi, and Brussels sprouts are also in that group. They are all high in soluble fiber, their vitamin content is high, and their antioxidant capacity is spectacular.

Scientists are now able to measure the antioxidant power of a substance. This measure is called the ORAC (oxygen radical absorbance capacity). Cruciferous vegetables contain phytonutrients called glucosinates, sulforaphane, and indoles. These compounds have cancer-fighting capabilities, fight inflammation, and support heart and joint health.

Kale has become one of my favorites, especially sautéed with garlic. It can also be used instead of lettuce in a salad. Be warned that kale does have a prominent taste, owing to PTC, a substance that people with a specific "taste gene" find distasteful. If you do like kale, you should feel great knowing that you are enjoying a unique taste and a powerful antioxidant with an ORAC of 1,770! That is a whopping dose of antioxidant power. It is well known that many vitamins, including vitamin C and vitamin E, are effective antioxidants.

CINNAMON AND APPLES

Is there anyone who doesn't love cinnamon sprinkled over baked apples? Of course there is, but I surely am not that person! I love the aroma of cinnamon and apples, and when I found out about the incredible anti-inflammatory value of cinnamon, I immediately stocked my cupboard. I may have been a bit impetuous, because cinnamon is anything but straightforward. There are several varieties of cinnamon, including cassia (Chinese) and zeylanicum (true cinnamon). Cassia has a stronger flavor and has a deep red-brown color, whereas zeylanicum has a lighter brown color. Zeylanicum is preferred for use in sweets by many confectioners, but cassia is sometimes used because it is less expensive.

The flavor and aroma of cinnamon bark come from its essential oil. The mouthwatering component of the oil, representing about 60 percent by volume, is cinnamaldehyde (CA). CA is the component teeming with health benefits (antitumor, antidiabetic, anti-inflammatory) and, unfortunately, potential toxicity. Warnings about toxicity have been sounded with another component in cassia, coumarin, which can have a toxic effect on the liver.

Patents are pending on hydroxycinnamaldehyde (HCA) derivatives to treat various cancers. Studies have shown two cinnamon derivatives to be potent anti-inflammatories. They can block NFkB through at least three different pathways! As a result of the NFkB blockade and cinnamon's delicious taste, your joints will love this aromatic spice as much as your palate. Cinnamon is an exceptional nutraceutical, but there is uncertainty about the appropriate dosage. Sprinkle it here and there, but it's not part of the daily supplement plan, because of its potential side effects. While it is tempting to include cinnamon in our daily plan, in larger doses as a supplement, I'm always extremely cautious about side effects, especially when it comes to the liver, so use it as a seasoning with confidence and in abundance, but we'll hold off on supplementation. I'll keep you abreast of the news about cinnamon via the healthyjointsforlife.com website and will let you know if I feel I can loosen my restrictions on cinnamon as a supplement.

WITHOUT VANILLIN THERE'D BE NO CHOCOLATE

Vanillin is a component of the vanilla bean. In fact, it imparts the flavor and aroma to the bean. Vanillin can be produced synthetically or naturally. The natural way is quite complex. The pods of the vanilla planifolia plant are harvested and subsequently blanched, sunned, sweated, and dried. This process takes several months and is costly—some forty times the cost of making synthetic vanillin. My favorite fact about vanillin, derived from vanilla, is that it is used to make chocolate. When I first learned that fact, I had never heard of anything so contradictory in my whole life. Imagine that 75 percent of the world's supply of vanillin is used to make chocolate ice cream.

If your household is like mine, the gals like chocolate ice cream and the guys like vanilla. Truth be told, I like just about any kind of ice cream! Vanillin is also used in perfumes and in some chemicals to hide unpleasant scents. All this flavoring and aroma should not hide the fact that in 2007 Murakami showed that vanillin inhibited NFkB activation and the inflammation related COX-2 gene expression in murine macrophages, a type of white blood cell that populates the synovium of joints. This is extremely important because the COX-2 enzyme is responsible for activating the inflammatory pathway and if it does so in the joint synovium, watch out for joint pain! Vanillin joins the indulgent food flavorings of our joint-healthy lifestyle.

COCOA

Any fellow chocoholics will be pleased to hear that there is fantastic news about research on cocoa. Cocoa helps prevent inflammation and thus is beneficial for joint health, and it should be part of a healthy cancer-prevention lifestyle, as well. Studies (Hooper 2008; Lee 2006; Rimbach 2009) have shown that components called polyphenols, extracted from regular cocoa powder, are quite joint healthy. Naturally, the sugar component of chocolate is proinflammatory, but unsweetened cocoa can be sweetened with Truvia to make delightful hot chocolate and homemade chocolate sweets. If you want to indulge in a small amount of chocolate, try dark chocolate, as it has the highest concentration of the good stuff. Milk chocolate is not as beneficial, because the concentration of cocoa is not as high and it contains a substantial amount of sugar.

BLACKBERRIES FOR EVERYONE

If you mention the word *blackberry* to people, they are more likely to think of a smartphone rather than a delicious bramble fruit. We need to change that, because blackberries have an ORAC of 5,347 per one hundred grams, which is extremely high among fruits. This ORAC is perhaps mainly due to blackberries' anthocyanidin content. Although they have never been formally tested, they are thought to have a low glycemic index, one similar to other berries. They are also teeming with vitamins, including vitamin C, vitamin K, and folate.

Italian researchers (Pergola 2006) have discovered that cyanidin-3-o-glucoside extracted from blackberries can inhibit NFkB. Blackberries are an excellent dessert choice for a healthy-joint lifestyle. Add a dollop of whipped cream to blackberries and you have an absolutely wonderful dessert. Try dipping blackberries into Truvia-sweetened dark chocolate for a delicious treat.

MANGOSTEEN: A DELIGHTFUL DRINK

The mangosteen tree *(Garcinia mangostana)* bears a two- to three-inch joint-healthy fruit full of antioxidants, including anthocyanidins, procyanidins, and xanthines. Gamma-mangostin, from the fruit hull, was shown to suppress NFkB and COX-2 gene transcription. Alpha- and gamma-mangostin may also inhibit the creation of "bad" prostaglandin E2 from arachidonic acid (see Devi 2007; Hung 2009; Nakatani 2002, 2004). Many sources recommend drinking one to three ounces of mangosteen juice per day, but one study comparing doses reported that eighteen ounces were necessary to have a substantial effect on inflammatory marker C-reactive protein. Mangosteen juice is expensive, but you can find it at Costco. Drinking eighteen ounces per day may strain your wallet, but a few delicious ounces of mangosteen juice, as a shot over ice, are delicious and joint healthy. Delicious and healthy, now, that's a dynamic duo!

***

Of course, eating healthfully is great. In subsequent chapters we'll discuss suggested meals in much greater detail. But sometimes, your body needs an extra boost that it can't get from fresh foods and vegetables. Supplements can be an excellent way to support your joints and the overall health of your body.

CHAPTER 4

SUPPORT:
Supplements

AS SCIENTIFIC RESEARCH MOUNTS, MAINSTREAM MEDICINE IS slowly recognizing and accepting the value of supplements. The long-held doubt, misunderstanding, and underestimation of the significance of their roles is slowly eroding in the medical community. The "Green Revolution" in the United States is a symbol of a nation becoming more receptive to the healthy wonders of nature. Lab and clinical studies are providing convincing evidence of the important roles for supplements in health. The previous lack of sufficient and specific scientific studies led mainstream medicine to be skeptical of teaching young doctors about supplements.

This chapter will address supplements that have been shown to be joint healthy. I will tell you about the risks associated with some supplements so you will understand why I don't recommend them. I'm going to direct you to my own research on my "stack" of supplements that have helped so many of my patients. (For those of you not familiar with bodybuilding lingo, a *stack* refers to a group of supplements taken together.) In this chapter I will briefly point out the research that got me interested in various supplements and will direct you to Appendix I for a more detailed discussion of the scientific research. I will also show you the synergistic benefit of taking these supplements in combination. To illustrate the effectiveness of these supplements, I will introduce you to a few patients along the way, showing you real patients, real arthritis, and real results.

SUPPLEMENTS, VITAMINS, MINERALS, AND MORE

When it comes to supplements, vitamins, minerals, nutraceuticals, and phytonutrients, the terminology can be confusing, so let me explain. A supplement is a relatively generic term referring to anything taken in addition to your diet. Any vitamin, mineral, nutraceutical or phytonutrient ingested in addition to your diet is a supplement. I'm sure all of you have heard of vitamins, but you probably don't know exactly what they are. Vitamins are not magic pills; they simply function as cofactors, or enzymes, in critical chemical reactions. You may recall that an enzyme speeds up a chemical reaction. For example, vitamin C is an enzyme used in the chemical reaction making collagen an important component of cartilage, ligaments, and tendons. Here's where it gets a little confusing. A vitamin is a supplement, but not all supplements are vitamins. Vitamin C in pill form is a vitamin that we take as a supplement to our diet. Calcium is an example of a mineral supplement. (Mineral? Think of a solid uniform crystal/rock.) It's a supplement but not a vitamin. Joint-healthy supplements, like curcumin, grape seed extract, pomegranate, green tea, and others, are not vitamins or minerals. Rather, they are nutraceuticals, purified natural food sources taken as a supplement. (The term nutraceutical derives from nutrition and pharmaceutical.) Supplements can also be called phytonutrients if they are derived from plants. Green tea is a natural food source, so it is a nutraceutical and, it is derived from a plant, so it is also a phytonutrient.

Various plant sources boast a plentiful amount of minerals, so minerals are contained in phytonutrients. Minerals are also contained in nutraceuticals. Magnesium, calcium, and selenium are examples of minerals.

For clarity I've separated the following sections into vitamins and "other" supplements.

SUPPLEMENTS AND THE SCIENTIFIC DATA

I am by nature a skeptic. As a physician, I want to see serious substantiation of drugs I prescribe or anything I recommend. The discussions that follow will briefly mention the science behind the supplements that I recommend; if you want more detailed information, please see Appendix I. Please also refer to the bibliography at the end of the book as well as a more extensive bibliography that can be found at www.healthyjointsforlife.com.

VITAMINS I RECOMMEND

The vitamins and other supplements I recommend pack a powerful punch when it comes to battling NFkB and, in turn, inflammation. As you know from the discussion of joint-healthy food in Chapter 3, there are many delicious natural sources for joint-friendly vitamins and minerals. However, it is difficult to get the full spectrum of joint-healthy nutrients in sufficient doses through diet alone, so supplementation is necessary.

TAKING YOUR VITAMINS AND OTHER SUPPLEMENTS

Water soluble means that the vitamin or supplement will dissolve in water, while *fat soluble* means it will dissolve in fat. This important distinction determines how you take a vitamin or supplement. You should take a fat-soluble vitamin or supplement with food (fat) to help absorption. Water-soluble vitamins or supplements can be taken with water and will be absorbed.

BIOAVAILABILITY

Supplements are of no value if they are not well absorbed into the body through the gastrointestinal system. Bioavailability is the medical term used to describe the body's ability to absorb a supplement and then have all its wonderful properties available for the body's cells to utilize. Many, if not most, supplements have limited bioavailability. Green tea, curcumin, grape seed extract, and silymarin, among others, are examples of supplements that have limited bioavailability. Sometimes, even when the supplement is absorbed, it gets conjugated or inactivated by the body. Scientists are therefore working on ways to improve supplements' absorption and to counteract their inactivation. For example, I am impressed with a patented process called phytosome (Kidd 2009). This is a process where a plant nutrient like curcumin, which is rather poorly absorbed, is bonded to phosphatidylcholine (PC), an emulsifying agent. This process allows the curcumin to be absorbed more efficiently, increasing its bioavailability by at least threefold. Other companies are using particle size to improve absorption. Nanotechnology generates particles as small as 1 to 2 microns! I mention these bioavailability techniques because you will undoubtedly encounter them when you buy your supplements. Claims about increased absorption need to be viewed critically and financially, because something that is absorbed two times as well may be four times as expensive.

A WORD TO THE WISE

Before adding any supplements to your diet, please consult with your doctor. Some dietary supplements may interact unfavorably with prescription and over-the-counter medications, can cause allergic reactions, or have other side effects. In the descriptions below, I will note significant side effects or potential drug interactions, but this list is by no means exhaustive. If no side effects are noted, it means that most people tolerate the supplement.

THE HEISMAN TROPHY
AND MY FIRST "VITAMINS"

During my college football days we didn't know that much about supplements. Let me tell you about my first experience with vitamins. If you are a college football fan, then you know about the Heisman Trophy, given each year to the most outstanding college football player in our great nation. It is on a pedestal higher than that of any other trophy, is certainly the most celebrated award in college football, and is the most coveted award in all of collegiate sports. Jay Berwanger won the first Heisman Trophy in 1935, and in 1936 and 1937 Yale football players Larry Kelley and Clint Frank were the recipients of the prestigious award. It is amazing to think that for two consecutive years Yale football players won the most coveted award in college sports. The horizon of college football has certainly changed. No other Yale player has ever won the Heisman. In fact, in the past seventy-three years only two Yale players have finished in the top ten of Heisman voting, Brian Dowling, aka BD, of *Doonesbury* cartoon fame, in 1969, and, well, me in 1982.

I bring up this subject because of a great memory I have of the last game of my college football career. And it happened to be the first time I ever took vitamins. We were playing Harvard on an unusually hot November day, and it was an amazing first half. Harvard was visiting us in New Haven, hoping for an upset. We were not about to let that happen. It was an incredibly intense game, full of punishing hits, and overlaid with the reality that it was the last football game of any sort for nearly all the seniors on both sides of the ball field. There would be no NFL for all but a few. The intensity level reflected that sense of urgency. With only one minute left in the first half, I caught a jailbreak screen pass and ran thirty-eight yards for a touchdown. Immediately, seventy-six thousand fans jumped out of their seats in either triumph or disgust. The Harvard team limped into halftime, trailing 14–0, but they were far from giving up.

I was feeling the intensity, as well. I was totally overheated and near exhaustion. I needed help. Our halftime room was like a cave underneath the stadium. The floor was a smooth, cool concrete, and the trainers attempted to cool me down by completely stripping me out of my uniform and laying me on the concrete floor with ice bags on my thighs, forehead, and abdomen. They made me drink plenty of water, and following the old belief, I swallowed a handful of salt tablets, "vitamins," as my teammates called them. I'd never considered taking salt pills before, but the prevailing thought was that they would keep my muscles from cramping up. Taking salt pills when overheated doesn't make any sense, and they most definitely are not vitamins, either! Me on the floor, covered in ice bags and swallowing salt pills, wasn't a pretty sight.

The halftime room had two doors, one that led to the field and another that led to the concourse outside the stadium, where all the fans collected to go to the concession stands. As I lay there with steam coming off me, the concourse door opened. Fans looked into the room, equally snickering and gasping at my mostly naked body steaming on the cool concrete floor. Then two elderly gentlemen guided by police officers stepped into the room. Because I was only eight feet in front of the door, they had no choice but to literally step over me. One of the elderly gentlemen looked down at me, lifted his leg and dropped one of his shoulders in a caricature of the Heisman Trophy pose, and said to me and the team, "Great game, fellas. I'm Larry Kelley, and this is Clint Frank." Clint Frank pulled on Larry Kelley's shirt after he stepped over me and said, "That's Diana, isn't it? He looks hot enough to fry an egg on 'im. Hope that ice gets him cooled down for the second half. And close that darn door. You'll scare the women." Turns out the two Yale greats were donating their Heisman Trophies to Yale and were passing through the room for the ceremony.

Without a doubt, that moment will remain my most unforgettable halftime memory, and it represents my introduction to the world of vitamins. Clearly, the vitamins I am about to recommend for joint health make much more sense than my salt pills. And they are all substantiated by research and clinical success. By the way, that day we beat Harvard 28–0 and captured the Ivy title. (My mother would be cringing right now, because she always said, "SPS, self-praise stinks.") It was a great way for all the Yale seniors to end their collegiate careers.

ANTI-INFLAMMATORY VITAMINS

My recommendations for anti-inflammatory vitamins include:

- Carotenoids (lutein and astaxanthin)
- Vitamin B_6

- Vitamin C
- Vitamin D
- Vitamin E (specifically a subclass of vitamin E called gamma-tocotrienol)

ALL IN GOOD MEASURE

Vitamins are measured in various ways. When you look at a bottle, you may see the abbreviations *mg* or *IU*. A milligram (mg) is a measure of mass or weight, whereas an international unit (IU) is an arbitrary unit of chemical activity defined by the WHO Expert Committee on Biological Standardization. It's important to know that 2000 mg does not equal 2000 IU.

CAROTENOIDS: LUTEIN AND ASTAXANTHIN

Lutein and astaxanthin are antioxidants from the carotenoid family that are very joint healthy. Technically they aren't vitamins but because they are closely associated with vitamin A I've included them here.

Lutein is from the carotene subgroup, and astaxanthin from the xanthophyll subgroup. Lutein can be found in green leafy vegetables, such as spinach and kale, while astaxanthin is found in salmon, micro algae, krill, and Arctic shrimp.

I associate anything from the carotenes with vitamin A, and I need to tell you that vitamin A has a checkered reputation in orthopedic circles. Some readers taking vitamin A (aka retinol) for eye (retina) health may have heard that excessive levels of vitamin A can lead to weak bones and fractures, especially if vitamin D levels are low. Vitamin A suppresses bone-forming cells, called osteoblasts, and activates bone-dissolving cells, called osteoclasts. Careful monitoring of daily supplementation of vitamin A is strongly recommended. This is why patients taking vitamin A concern orthopedic surgeons.

To protect your bones, instead of supplementing with vitamin A, experts say it is safer to supplement with beta-carotene, another member of the carotenoid family found in yellow and orange fruits, such as cantaloupe, mangos, and papayas; in root vegetables, such as yams and carrots; and in leafy green vegetables, such as kale and spinach. Beta-carotene can be converted to vitamin A by enzymes, but experts maintain that the body's own feedback mechanisms will prevent the overproduction of vitamin A. It sounds good, but I think it is better to be safe than sorry, and I'd like you to avoid any carotenoid that can be converted into vitamin A. The good news about astaxanthin and lutein is that the body cannot convert either of them into vitamin A, so neither is potentially dangerous for your bones. We don't have to worry about feedback mechanisms functioning optimally. There are no enzymes to convert either nutrient into vitamin A.

I like both of these carotenoids because of their impact on NFkB and their amazing antioxidant power. Astaxanthin is one hundred times as strong an antioxidant as vitamin E and is more potent than lutein, as well. Astaxanthin is also cool because it is the molecule responsible for the red/orange color shrimp and lobster acquire when they are cooked.

RECOMMENDED DAILY DOSAGE	
Lutein	10-40 mg
Astaxanthin	2-4 mg

VITAMIN B$_6$

Vitamin B$_6$ is an extremely important and busy enzyme that is involved in how amino acids, fats, and sugar are processed by the body to produce energy. Its suppressing effect on NFkB makes it joint healthy.

Vitamin B_6 plays an essential role in the production of chemicals that are important in the proper functioning of the body. The neurotransmitters (chemical messengers that nerves secrete) serotonin, GABA, and dopamine are all made from amino acids under the enzymatic guidance of vitamin B_6. Vitamin B_6 also facilitates the production of ceramides, incredibly important fatty molecules made of sphingosine and a fatty acid, which represent a large component of the lipid bilayer, or cell membrane. Ceramide is also significant as a signaling messenger for cell death. Ceramide released from the cell membrane can signal the cell to start the cascade toward cell death, an extremely important process in preventing the formation of inflammation and cancers.

The role of vitamin B_6 in necessary cell death is an indirect means by which it helps fight cancer. Vitamin B_6 is also pivotal in the conversion of amino acids into glucose in a process called gluconeogenesis (gluco = sugar, neo = new, genesis = production; the production of new sugar), as well as in the breakdown of liver glycogen into glucose (remember that the body uses glucose as fuel). With the ability to perform all of those functions, I'd call vitamin B_6 one versatile vitamin.

It is also important to take a vitamin B complex containing all the B vitamins because the B vitamins are codependent, meaning they work together. B_6 is like the quarterback, and the other Bs help to protect the quarterback, like the offensive linemen on a football team. If you want your B_6 to work well, then you need to take the other Bs—thiamine (B_1, 1.1–1.2 mg/d), riboflavin (B_2, 1.1–1.3 mg/d), niacin (B_3, 14–16 mg/d), pantothenic acid (B_5, 5 mg/d), biotin (B_7, 30 ug/d), folate (B_9, 400 ug/d), and cobalamin (B_{12}, 2.4 ug/d)—and choline (425–550 mg/d), which is usually grouped with the B vitamins. All these B vitamins should be on your team, and at minimum they should be taken according to United States Department of Agriculture (USDA) recommendations.

RECOMMENDED DAILY DOSAGE	
Vitamin B$_6$	10-20 mg
Vitamin B complex	at above dosages

Potential side effects: Doses of B$_6$ over 200 mg/day can have serious neurological side effects, like hand or foot numbness or even difficulty walking, so be careful about how much B$_6$ you are taking.

VITAMIN C

Vitamin C is necessary for collagen formation, which is essential for many tissues, including skin, ligaments, and cartilage. Hydroxyl groups (OH groups) are added to collagen under the vigilant watch of vitamin C. The addition of OH groups allows collagen to form its three-dimensional helix shape. Vitamin C is essential for type II collagen synthesis (a pivotal type for joint cartilage) and is especially important for joint health. If you want to ensure an appropriate supply of healthy type II collagen for your ligaments and articular cartilage, then take vitamin C.

In 2003 Korean investigators showed that vitamin C can inhibit NFkB and thereby down-regulates TNF-alpha, another one of those dreaded messengers of inflammation. Most animals and plants can make vitamin C from glucose, but guinea pigs, monkeys, apes, humans, and some birds cannot, because they lack the enzyme gulonolactone oxidase. Therefore we humans must get vitamin C either through the food we eat or by taking a supplement.

IF YOU DON'T HAVE ENOUGH C AT SEA

Lack of vitamin C can lead to a fatal disease known as scurvy. Through the ages it was often the cause of death for sailors on long voyages. With no foods providing vitamin C while they were at sea, sailors would develop

continued

bleeding gums and skin spots and wounds, and they would ultimately die. While the consumption of citrus fruits was described hundreds of years ago as the way to prevent and cure scurvy, the disease wasn't understood until 1932, when a lack of vitamin C was identified as the culprit. Having citrus fruit, which provided the necessary vitamin C, as part of their diet rescued the sailors from this disease.

There are many types of vitamin C on the market. Vitamin C is ascorbic acid and as the word *acid* implies, it may be upsetting to the stomach. Some of my patients feel that Ester-C, a variety of vitamin C buffered with calcium, is easier on the stomach, and it may be more quickly absorbed. PureWay-C, a recently developed vitamin C–lipid metabolite, may be the most quickly absorbed vitamin C preparation available presently. Individual doses greater than 500 mg are not well absorbed, so take 500 mg two times per day.

RECOMMENDED DAILY DOSAGE
500 mg 2 times per day
(Note that the USDA recommends less than 100 mg/day. I feel that this is an inadequate amount.)

VITAMIN D

Vitamin D plays a pivotal role in bone health as it facilitates calcium absorption from the GI tract. Because it supports better absorption, normal blood levels of calcium are easier to maintain. Parathyroid hormone, which resorbs calcium from bone, is suppressed by vitamin D. This supports bone strength. Vitamin D also plays an important role in subduing joint inflammation by inhibiting NFkB in specialized white blood cells. Vitamin D has previously little-recognized roles in general immune function, mood control, muscle strength, athletic performance, insulin regulation, blood pressure control, heart health, and cancer protection.

You can get vitamin D from supplementation or sunlight exposure. Fortunately, supplements are inexpensive and sunlight is free! There are several forms of vitamin D which I fully describe in Appendix I under the vitamin D subheading. Suffice it to say that the supplement you want to take is vitamin D_3 (cholecalciferol). Previously, it was felt that 35 ng/ml was a sufficient blood level of the vitamin D metabolite 25-hydroxy vitamin D, but now it is felt that 50 ng/ml is appropriate. The current USDA recommendation for vitamin D_3 is 400 IU, but this amount of vitamin D_3 appears insufficient to maintain 50 ng/ml levels. Studies showing that up to 60 percent of females and 50 percent of males are vitamin D deficient indicate that higher levels of supplementation are necessary. Research from Creighton University recommends 5000 IU/day, more than twelve times the current recommendations.

Recognizing the pandemic nature of vitamin D deficiency, the Vitamin D Council recommendation for higher baseline vitamin D levels, and the Creighton University research, I, too, recommend 5000 IU/day of vitamin D_3 monitored by blood levels of 25-hydroxy vitamin D. Vitamin D toxicity is rare, so the ingestion of supplements is quite safe. Monitoring blood levels of vitamin D is recommended to determine subtherapeutic low levels as much as higher levels. Note that patient weight will influence the amount of vitamin D necessary to achieve appropriate levels.

If you are on the fence as to whether to take vitamin D, you might consider a study that showed that the chromosomes of women with low vitamin D levels are five years "older" than those of women with higher vitamin D levels.

RECOMMENDED DAILY DOSAGE
A baseline 25-hydroxy vitamin D blood level should be obtained. This is determined by a simple blood test.
Ten to twenty minutes of sunlight (if fair skinned; more time if darker skinned). Without that level of sun exposure, the dose is dependent on baseline blood level. Depending on body weight 2000–5000 IU of vitamin D_3 is necessary to maintain 50 ng/ml blood level.
Potential side effects: Vitamin D_3 is quite safe but supplementing at extremely high doses is not recommended and can cause heart arrhythmias, nausea, vomiting, and kidney failure. (See Appendix I for more information.)

VITAMIN E

Vitamin E is not a single vitamin, but a family of fat-soluble vitamins. They are generally divided into tocopherols and tocotrienols. I know those names can be confusing, but it is important to know them because most vitamin E supplements that you can purchase are tocopherols, which are important for joint health, but only in a supporting role. The most joint-healthy subclass of vitamin E is the tocotrienols, gamma-tocotrienol being the specific type of vitamin E that you want for joint health. If you purchase "regular" vitamin E, you won't be getting the appropriate vitamin E mixture to help your joints. Gamma-tocotrienol is an anti-inflammatory and a potent inhibitor of NFkB. As an additional benefit, it also helps control cholesterol production, so it is heart-healthy, too!

Foods containing vitamin E include vegetable oils, nuts, seeds, and whole grains. Vitamin E can also be found in green leafy vegetables and tomatoes.

RECOMMENDED DAILY DOSAGE
Tocotrienols: gamma- 15 mg, alpha- and delta- 15 mg or less. Tocopherols: 100 IU 1x/day of a full-spectrum blend. (Tocotrienols are measured in mg, and tocopherols in IU.) Check the label to ensure you are getting the correct amounts.
Potential side effects: Can cause bleeding. Check with your doctor if you are taking anticoagulants.

SUPPLEMENTS...BEYOND VITAMINS

Having discussed vitamins, the following section will discuss mineral, oil, and plant supplements that are exceptionally joint healthy.

ANTI-INFLAMMATORY SUPPLEMENTS

My recommendations for anti-inflammatory supplements include:

- Calcium
- Omega-3 Fatty Acids
- Grape Seed Extract
- Resveratrol
- Curcumin
- Boswellia
- Pomegranate
- Ginger
- Green Tea
- Glucosamine and Chondroitin
- Licorice
- N-Acetyl Cysteine (NAC)
- Silymarin

CALCIUM

Maintaining bone strength is vital to joint health. Magnesium, potassium, phosphorous, vitamins B, C, D, and K, and carotenoids are all important for bone structure, but calcium may be the most important. Ninety-nine percent of body calcium is stored in the bones, and the other 1 percent is of vital importance for various body functions, such as muscle contraction (remember, the heart is a muscle) and nerve conduction. This means that calcium is very important not only for bone strength but also for heart and brain function.

The distribution of calcium throughout the body needs to be very specifically monitored. Although representing a small fraction of total body calcium, the blood calcium level must be held in precise balance, or critical events, like heart arrhythmias, occur. This balance has a major effect on bone strength, because as blood calcium levels drop, parathyroid hormone increases, removing calcium from bone to boost blood calcium. Too much calcium removed from the bones results in osteoporosis (the weakening of bones).

We know from various studies (Rodríguez-Rodríguez 2010; Bailey 2010; Ma 2007; Poliquin 2009; Garriguet 2011; Flynn 2003) that many subgroups of the population don't get enough calcium. The elderly, especially elderly women, and adolescent females are particularly deficient. While inadequate intake does not lead to immediate bone weakening (osteoporosis), it can be a devastating problem over time. Calcium is an amazing mineral. Those of us concerned with joint health and obesity are particularly interested in studies that link increased calcium intake to weight loss (Rodríguez-Rodríguez 2010).

Vitamin D helps calcium get absorbed in the GI tract, so vitamin D and calcium must be taken together to insure that bone and body calcium levels are maintained. Bailey showed that 42 percent of the U.S. population take calcium supplements, but only 12 percent of those seventy-one years old or older meet adequate intake for calcium. This tells us that although people may be taking calcium supplements, they may not be taking sufficient quantities or their vitamin D levels are so low that the calcium isn't being absorbed into the body.

Although calcium does not reduce inflammation, I recommend that you take calcium primarily to fortify your bones, to prevent bone fractures and collapse, as well as to support other important body functions.

High-protein diets, which I recommend in this book, are known to be acidic and to increase urinary calcium elimination. That has led many experts in nutrition to assume that high-protein diets are bad for your bones. Many physicians, and even a few patients, have specifically asked me about this very issue, so it is very important that I clarify this. Epidemiological studies have shown that long-term high-protein diets increase bone mineral density. While it is true that urinary calcium elimination increases, calcium absorption in the intestine is increased, and parathyroid hormone, which removes calcium from the bones, is suppressed. The net effect is increased bone mineral density (Cao 2010). If you want to have strong bones, take calcium and vitamin D. Dairy products are great sources of calcium, as are almonds, collard greens, kale, spinach, soybeans, sardines, and salmon.

In addition, exercise maintains strong bones by indirectly keeping calcium in the bones. To help battle osteoporosis by maintaining bone calcium, make sure that your exercise is weight bearing, varied, and stressful intermittently (Borer 2005). (See Chapter 5 on exercise.)

The NIH Office of Dietary Supplements recommends:

AGE	MALE	FEMALE	PREGNANT	LACTATING
0–6 months*	200 mg	200 mg		
7–12 months*	260 mg	260 mg		
1–3 years	700 mg	700 mg		

continued

AGE	MALE	FEMALE	PREGNANT	LACTATING
4–8 years	1000 mg	1000 mg		
9–13 years	1300 mg	1300 mg		
14–18 years	1300 mg	1300 mg	1300 mg	1300 mg
19–50 years	1000 mg	1000 mg	1000 mg	1000 mg
51–70 years	1000 mg	1200 mg		
71+ years	1200 mg	1200 mg		

* Adequate Intake (AI)

From http://ods.od.nih.gov/factsheets/Calcium-HealthProfessional/#h2

Patients frequently ask me what type of calcium they should purchase: chelated (calcium attached to an amino acid or an organic molecule, i.e., a carbon-containing molecule) versus non-chelated. There remains significant debate about the type of calcium that is best absorbed. Harvey (1988) showed that calcium citrate, considered a chelated calcium, is better absorbed than non-chelated calcium carbonate, whereas Heaney (1999) found that both were absorbed equally. Some say that non-chelated calcium simply becomes chelated in the gut, completely explaining Heaney's results. I say, go for the chelated variety.

Recent studies have shown a concerning relationship between heart attacks, strokes, and calcium supplementation (Li 2012). Study participants on calcium supplementation had a significantly increased risk of heart attacks and strokes, while high dietary intake of calcium was not associated with an increased risk of heart attacks or strokes. This presents an obvious dilemma: bone health versus heart health. I would recommend modifying calcium supplementation and increasing dietary intake as the safest method of dealing with calcium intake. For example, if you should be taking 1000 mg of calcium daily, then it would be prudent to get the majority of that intake from diet. You'll need to determine how much calcium you get from your diet and supplement only that amount necessary to attain 1000 mg.

Until the cardiovascular risk dilemma is settled, I would not exceed supplementation of more than 250 mg two times per day. Consult your cardiologist for further information and discussion.

RECOMMENDED DAILY DOSAGE

Get most of your recommended daily calcium from food. Consult your cardiologist, but do not exceed supplementation of 500 mg maximum. Take 250 mg 2 times per day, depending on estimated dietary intake of calcium. (See above text for foods containing calcium.)

Potential side effects: See above cardiovascular side effects. People with kidney disease should observe caution, as calcium levels can rise dangerously. Can cause gastrointestinal upset, headache, or constipation. Not to be taken with alendronate (Fosamax), antacids that contain aluminum (Maalox), beta-blockers (Tenormin, Inderal, Toprol-XL, Lopressor), calcium channel blockers (verapamil, diltiazem, amlodipine), digoxin, diuretics (Lasix, hydrochlorothiazide), iron, antiseizure medications (Dilantin, phenobarbital), or antibiotics (Cipro, tetracycline).

OMEGA-3 FATTY ACIDS

Taking omega-3 fatty acids is good for joint health. Yes, you read correctly—these fats taken daily will help you to remain healthy. Omega-3s are very healthy fats that are found in sardines, mackerel, salmon, swordfish, krill, flaxseed, hemp, grass-fed beef, and non-corn-fed chicken eggs. Omega-3s can help with asthma and heart disease, and are great for joint health. There are several omega-3 fatty acids. The omega-3s I recommend are DHA (docosohexanoic acid) and EPA (eicosapentnoic acid). A quick look at Appendix I will show how these wonderfully joint-healthy omega-3 fatty acids work. I love the effect DHA has on resolvin synthesis and the effect EPA has on anti-inflammatory prostaglandin synthesis.

Dozens of studies from the United States, Europe, and the Far East have all demonstrated the positive effects of omega-3s on

NFkB and the anti-inflammatory pathways. Some of the studies have concentrated on the cardiac benefits or the anticancer effects of omega-3s, and others have established important implications for joint health. The results of these studies, and my knowledge of the anti-inflammatory pathways, prompted me to conduct a study of the benefits of omega-3s with my own patients. With great enthusiasm I started a trial in which I treated patients with various osteoarthritic joints solely with omega-3s. Many of those patients who agreed to be in the trial were concerned with the side effects of traditional non-steroidal anti-inflammatory medications (NSAIDs), like Celebrex, Motrin, and Naprosyn, so I considered omega-3s as an alternative treatment for them. You may not be aware that the side effects of NSAIDs, including bleeding ulcers, are responsible for 16,500 deaths per year in the United States, as well as billions of dollars in medical costs annually. It's no wonder why so many people want to avoid them if possible.

So that they could avoid NSAIDs and find a viable alternative for pain relief, I placed thirty patients on omega-3 supplementation over a three-month period. When the study first started, I was hopeful. After several positive results, I came to expect good news. In total, nearly 60 percent of patients reported improvements in their symptoms; some experienced mild improvement, and others more remarkable improvement.

RECOMMENDED DAILY DOSAGE
Omega-3 1000 mg 2 times per day with a minimum of DHA 300 mg and EPA 500 mg
Potential side effects: Diarrhea, stomach upset, repeating (regurgitation, burping), fish breath, blood thinning, or bleeding at higher doses.

GRAPE SEED EXTRACT

The grape seed contains proanthocyanidins (PACs), strings of epicatechin molecules that are closely related to the miracle molecule of green tea. PACs have the ability to help prevent damage to blood vessel walls, skin, tendons, cartilage, and muscle, so are considered joint healthy for tendons, cartilage, and muscle.

PACs can scavenge damaging free radicals fifty times better than vitamin C and twenty times better than vitamin E, making them even greater antioxidants. PACs also have the ability to prevent wrinkles!

BENEFITS OF THE GRAPE

The "French Paradox" is the term put forth to encapsulate the observation that despite their typically high-fat diet, the French are protected from heart disease because of red wine consumption. Since Serge Renaud introduced us to the French Paradox in 1992, the grape has been thoroughly analyzed. It has been determined that the secret to the grape's health benefits lies in its skin and seeds, as opposed to its sweet inner flesh.

RECOMMENDED DAILY DOSAGE
200 mg divided into morning and nighttime doses
Potential side effects: Can be a blood thinner. Has the potential to cause headache, nausea, as well as dry and itchy scalp.

RESVERATROL TO THE RESCUE

Resveratrol is the other extraordinary molecule in grapes that is joint healthy. Initially, it gained worldwide recognition as a life-span extender, as it was shown to extend the life expectancy of yeast, fruit flies, and fish. Pharmaceutical giant GlaxoSmithKline found the potential of this molecule so exciting that it bought resveratrol-based Sirtris Pharmaceuticals for 720 million dollars in 2008. Through the activation of the enzyme SIRT1 (Silent Information Regulator Two-1), resveratrol can inactivate NFkB, fight against inflammation, and facilitate metabolism (Milne 2007).

Resveratrol's potential, especially as a life-span extender, has been scrutinized by many. Questions about the original research, as well as subsequent falsification of research by another major resveratrol researcher, have many concerned (see Appendix I for further explanation). While a small portion of the research is questionable, the vast majority is supportive of resveratrol. I recommend resveratrol for joint health and have found it to be helpful to patients.

Joint pain as a result of taking resveratrol has been written about, but it appears that this occurs primarily in those people with low vitamin D levels. Resveratrol is not recommended for those with gout or for those on cholesterol-lowering statin drugs, like Lipitor; calcium channel blockers, like verapamil; or erectile dysfunction drugs, like Viagra. If you are taking any of these medications and also take resveratrol, you may experience increases in your medication blood levels.

Studies, including those by Majumdar, 2009, and Csaki, 2008, show promising synergistic effects between resveratrol and other supplements for joint arthritis, cancer prevention, and antiaging. We'll look into these claims and others for possible promising synergistic effects in the discussions of other supplements. I should warn you that resveratrol is expensive, about $1.25 per 250 mg for the more highly absorbed micronized varieties, but I think it will prove to be worth it.

RECOMMENDED DAILY DOSAGE
250 mg

Potential side effects: Not for use in pregnancy since it may affect the fetus. Not recommended for those with gout or those on cholesterol-lowering statin drugs, like Lipitor; calcium channel blockers, like verapamil; or erectile dysfunction drugs, like Viagra. You may experience nausea, diarrhea, joint aches, or Achilles tendinitis.

CURCUMIN

The enticing golden-yellow color of many South Asian curry dishes is from the spice turmeric *(Curcuma longa)*. The plant root and underground stem are ground up to make the pungent spice. The biologically active portion of turmeric, called curcumin, has been the subject of significant research recently, and it has been shown to be a potent anti-inflammatory. It has also been the subject of several cancer clinical trials.

Curcumin has inhibitory effects on NFkB and other inflammatory messengers! It is also a strong antioxidant and free radical scavenger. It can even trigger the production of glutathione, our body's most potent and dynamic antioxidant. Its specific effect on cartilage cells has received considerable attention. Many researchers are excited about its prospects in the treatment of osteoarthritis. As incredible as curcumin sounds, scientists are trying to make it even better by modifying its molecular structure (see Appendix I).

The big problem with curcumin is its bioavailability. Bioavailability refers to a substance's ease of absorption into the bloodstream. Curcumin is not soluble in water at the acidic pH of the stomach. When it is absorbed, it is transformed into curcumin-glucuronate or sulfate, which are both inactive. The idea, then, is to get it out of the stomach and into the small intestine, where the pH is better suited to absorption. Biocurcumax, otherwise known as BCM-95, in which curcumin is mixed with "oil of turmeric," does this. Studies show curcumin blood levels at six times that of regular curcumin when taken as biocurcumax. There are questions about how long the "regular" curcumin supplements stay in the blood before being transformed into the inactive form, curcumin-glucuronate or sulfate. The research on biocurcumax is very positive, revealing slower inactivation and prolonged blood levels.

Some suggest combining curcumin with coconut milk, chocolate, omega-3s, olive oil, DMSO (dimethyl sulfoxide, a solvent that is readily absorbed by the body and has anti-inflammatory effects by itself), or piperine (a component of black pepper that appears to interfere with drug breakdown and thereby increases bioavailability) to facilitate bioavailability.

Nanocurcumin is another high-tech preparation of curcumin that you will come across when buying curcumin. It encapsulates 50 nm (50×10^{-9} meters—that's really, really small) particles of curcumin in polymers that are soluble in water. This may help with absorption.

Biocurcumax/BCM-95 is the more highly absorbed form that I have the most experience with. I recommend taking it with omega-3s two times per day to try to further improve bioavailability.

Curcumin happens to be one of the supplements that is highly synergistic when combined with resveratrol. I find combining the two supplements an exciting strategy for battling joint pain (see Appendix I for the science).

RECOMMENDED DAILY DOSAGE
Biocurcumax 250–500 mg 2 times per day
Potential side effects: May sensitize skin to light and effect blood sugar levels.

MY PATIENT THERESA

Theresa was thirty-five years old when I first met her. She had three active children who dominated her life when she wasn't working a part-time job, trying to make ends meet. Between the job and shuttling the kids to their activities, she was eating at the rink or the ballpark, never exercising, and beginning to have terrible knee pain. When I met her, she weighed 165 pounds and was tired. She dreaded having to go up stairs or walk from the car to her office. She was convinced she needed surgery to overcome her knee pain. Her concerns led to a full workup, each test—X-rays, MRI, ultrasound, blood tests—coming back normal or darn close to it. Each time I told her that a test was normal, she doubted the result. She couldn't believe it. Luckily, she was a friend of my secretary, so she didn't leave me for a second opinion! If she had, I wonder if she might have ended up with an unnecessary knee surgery.

When the last test, an MRI, came back negative, I told her I could make her feel a lot better, but it would take an effort on her part. I introduced her to my program of joint-healthy nutrition, exercise, and supplements. I reached into my bag of motivating tricks and turned to her three sons, aged fourteen, eleven, and nine. I asked them if they thought mom could do it. I wasn't sure if they would be supportive and would give Theresa that bit of confidence that she needed, or if, as I have subsequently learned, they would do what a typical group of three young boys would do to their parent—irritate, infuriate. Well, those of you who have boys guessed right; they laughed at Mom and mocked her ability to change. That was all Theresa needed to be motivated to prove them wrong. Right in front of me she turned red, grimaced at them, and developed "the eye of the tiger." Six months later she had lost nearly

continued

thirty pounds and was exercising regularly, eating a joint-healthy diet, and taking a handful of supplements. She had a substantial reduction in pain, an abundance of energy, and the motivation to prove her kids wrong. The last time I saw her, I asked how she was doing, and she said, "I'm doing a lot better." Her eldest son added, "You look a lot better, too, Mom." It was the first time I saw her smile.

BOSWELLIA

In the Bible it is said that three wise men brought gold, frankincense, and myrrh to the baby Jesus. The scientific name of the tree from which frankincense is derived is *Boswellia*. There are several species of *Boswellia*, including those indigenous to Somalia *(B. carteri, B. papyrifera,* and *B. rivae)* and Ethiopia *(B. serrata)*. The resin of the tree contains boswellic acid, the chemically active part of boswellia, which, as you can probably guess, has anti-inflammatory effects. Boswellia with AKBA is most potent. Avoid beta-boswellic acid.

There are numerous animal studies of boswellia available for evaluation; however, two quality randomized, controlled studies were presented in the *Journal of Clinical Rheumatology* (Chopra 2004) and *PhytoMedicine* (Kimmatkar 2003). They evaluated ninety and thirty patients, respectively. Both of these studies showed effective symptomatic treatment of osteoarthritis with boswellia. The 2004 study also included other herbs in the tested formula.

An interesting study from the University of Ulm in Germany (Sterk 2004) found that taking boswellia with a high-fat meal led to a several-fold increase in plasma concentrations. This may indicate that similar to curcumin, boswellia should be taken with omega-3 fatty acids. Neither of these human studies indicated toxicity. As an added bonus, boswellia reduces cholesterol levels. I am most familiar with BosPure boswellia which has high AKBA content and no beta-boswellic acid.

RECOMMENDED DAILY DOSAGE
300 mg 2 times per day
Potential side effects: Can cause stomach upset and abdominal bloating. Not for use by pregnant women. Not to be combined with cancer-treating medications, antifungal medications, or cholesterol-lowering medications.

POMEGRANATE

I can vividly recall eating pomegranates as a kid, because of the bright red staining on my hands. That staining on our couch convinced my mother that pomegranates weren't for us. They disappeared from our household, and for thirty years I didn't see or hear of them again. Five years ago at a neighborhood party, I was reintroduced to pomegranates—this time in a martini! I'll simply tell you that it was a great party and leave it at that.

Pomegranates seem to have made a recent resurgence, and I couldn't be happier. I love the flavor, and I am intrigued by the Case Western Reserve University study (Ahmed 2005) that showed that pomegranate fruit extract protected cartilage from arthritic breakdown. NFkB was inhibited, and cartilage cells were prevented from excreting the battery acid–like, destructive MMPs that eat away the cartilage Jell-O-like ECM. Pomegranate juice is a promising supplement for those with osteoarthritis.

RECOMMENDED DAILY DOSAGE
250–500 mg 2 times per day
Potential side effects: May cause allergic reactions and stomach upset. May decrease blood pressure and may increase the effect of blood pressure medications. May increase levels of medicines metabolized by the liver, such as Elavil, Ultram, Prozac, Lasix, Vasotec, and Norvasc.

GINGER

Ginger comes from a plant closely related to turmeric. The root of the *Zingiber officinale* plant is sliced thinly to reveal a luscious pale yellow, fleshy delight that has powerful anti-inflammatory properties. When my family orders sushi, I always quickly grab my share of the pickled ginger. It goes quickly. It has a wonderful aroma and a mouthwatering taste. I say mouthwatering because it is a sialagogue, meaning it stimulates the production of saliva. Pickled ginger is excellent eaten alone, but I love fresh ginger as a flavoring for shrimp, chicken, and vegetables. You can combine it with citrus juices, like orange or lemon, for a delicious, refreshing drink on a hot day. Beware that pickled ginger does contain sugar so fresh is preferred for cooking.

Ginger has been extremely well researched in hundreds of osteoarthritis patients and has undergone significant bench research, as well (Ahmed 2008, 2000; Aktan 2006; Altman 2001). There are several studies supporting the use of ginger in treating joint inflammation. I discuss some of them in Appendix I. These studies include a double-blind, placebo-controlled study where two-thirds of patients with osteoarthritis responded favorably.

Ginger is not for people on blood thinners (it may further thin blood by inhibiting thromboxane, a component of the clotting process) or people with gallstones, as it promotes the production of bile, which is what forms stones (Skenderi 2003; Skidmore-Roth 2003; Karch 1999).

Ginger is an absolutely delicious spice when eaten fresh or it can be taken in pill form. Eat fresh ginger as much as you can, in addition to taking ginger as a supplement.

RECOMMENDED DAILY DOSAGE
500–1000 mg

Potential side effects: Do not take if you have gallstones. Can have a blood-thinning effect. If you are taking blood-thinning medications, such as Plavix or Coumadin, be careful of taking ginger with garlic or omega-3s. This can lead to dangerous bleeding.

GREEN TEA

I've loved green tea since my younger days, when my family went to the local Japanese restaurant and green tea would be poured into small porcelain cups. I remember my hands and my whole body warming up from the heat radiating from the porcelain.

In 1999 a Japanese study by Dulloo showed that 270 mg of epigallocatechin gallate (EGCG), the active component of green tea, separated in three doses, was thermogenic, meaning that EGCG is heat generating. The tea was warming me from the outside in and the inside out. All by itself, green tea speeds up metabolism and burns calories. The Japanese study specifically stated that by drinking the right amount of green tea (270 mg of EGCG), you would burn sixty-three calories per day without lifting a thumb! That may not sound like many calories, but burning sixty-three calories a day for over a year results in a loss of about six pounds of fat. Other studies done in 2007 (Nagao) and 2008 (Auvichayapat) showed similar results. When 583 mg of tea catechins (a component of green tea extract) were ingested, LDL "bad" cholesterol and blood pressure both decreased. Green tea extract, therefore, has cardiovascular benefits, as well.

There is great news, as well, for women over the age of sixty. Bone strength, referred to as bone mineral density (BMD), can be improved simply by drinking green tea. It may not be that the green tea increases BMD, as much as it lowers the rate at which BMD is decreasing. For example, in the Muraki 2007 study, tea drinkers lost 1.6 percent BMD over four years, while nondrinkers lost 4 percent.

Green tea has other orthopedic benefits. I am very excited about a 2009 study by Rasheed from the University of South Carolina School of Medicine showing that EGCG in green tea inhibits advanced glycation end products (AGEs), as well as TNF-alpha and MMP-13 in human cartilage cells. That's exactly what this doctor ordered!

EGCG blocks NFkB and twenty-nine other inflammatory proteins! It protects cartilage from collagen breakdown, so it is a great addition to any regimen for joint health (Akhtar 2011; Katiyar 2011). Brewed green tea is relaxing, especially when it is warm. The relaxation alone makes green tea worthwhile. I also like the fact that drinking green tea can be substituted for eating an unhealthy snack after dinner or while relaxing at night. (Don't drink it too close to bedtime, because the caffeine content is roughly 25 mg per eight ounces. Black tea contains approximately twice as much caffeine as green tea.) Each cup of green tea provides 20 to 35 mg of EGCG, so unless you are going to drink ten cups per day, you should consider supplementing. The great news is that green tea supplements are inexpensive, at less than fifteen cents per day! The positive effects on obesity, the cardiovascular system, and joint health make EGCG an absolute no-brainer.

RECOMMENDED DAILY DOSAGE

1 cup brewed green tea and at least 270 mg EGCG (split into two or three doses)

Potential side effects: Due to its caffeine content, can cause headache, insomnia, irregular heartbeat, dizziness, tremors, diarrhea, increased pressure in eyes (glaucoma), increased blood pressure, and liver disease. Not to be used in pregnancy, owing to caffeine's link to miscarriage.

GIUSEPPE AND THE BROCCOLI AND CAULIFLOWER

As a practicing orthopedic surgeon, there is no question that I am asked more frequently about glucosamine and chondroitin than about all other nutraceuticals combined. One of my favorite discussions was with a patient who asked about the "broccoli and cauliflower" stuff Costco was selling for joint pain. I had no idea what he was talking about until his wife pulled out a bottle of glucosamine and chondroitin. How he derived "broccoli and cauliflower" out of glucosamine and chondroitin, I don't know, but to this day I still smile thinking about our subsequent conversation.

"Giuseppe, it's a little controversial, but yes, I think there is good evidence that glucosamine and chondroitin can help your joint pain," I said.

"What you mean, Doc?" he said.

"I mean that glucosamine and chondroitin have been shown in many European studies and some American studies to help with joint pain," I reiterated.

"What do you mean, Doctor? Glucos and chondroit?" he said, getting irritated with me and the big words I was using.

"Giuseppe, glucosamine and chondroitin is the stuff in the bottle that your wife showed me a moment ago. Take it! I think it will help," I said.

"Oh, Doc, you mean the broccoli and cauliflower," he said.

"Yes," I said, succumbing to the futility of the situation. "Giuseppe, please take the broccoli and cauliflower. Please take it."

GLUCOSAMINE AND CHONDROITIN

There is some question both about the importance of supplementing with glucosamine and chondroitin, and about how well they work on relieving joint pain. Glucosamine is an important component of joint fluid and the sugar proteins of the cartilage Jell-O-like ECM, and chondroitin is an important component of another type of sugar protein of the cartilage Jell-O-like ECM. Both are extremely important for healthy joints. But just because they are components of the joint cartilage and synovial fluid doesn't necessarily mean that taking them is going to be helpful in alleviating pain or correcting damage.

Because patients frequently ask about glucosamine and chontroitin, I stay up to date on the research and literature so I can give them information they can use. When considering the research on glucosamine and chondroitin, I separate it into European studies and American studies. In general, the European studies are quite favorable, to the point where glucosamine and chondroitin are prescription drugs in Europe. The studies done in America are not as favorable. The largest American study, done through the National Institutes of Health in 2008 and called the Glucosamine/chondroitin Arthritis Intervention Trial (GAIT), evaluated 1,583 patients and concluded that, overall, glucosamine and chondroitin did *not* reduce pain compared to placebo. Further analysis of the patient population did show, however, that 79 percent of patients with *moderate to severe arthritis* did respond favorably. This is very important information to consider when determining who should be taking glucosamine and chondroitin to receive the benefit they can offer. A follow-up GAIT study by Sawitzke (2010) of 662 patients, over two years, further studied this subgroup and noted beneficial but not significant trends for glucosamine as well as the prescription NSAID, Celebrex.

A 2008 Swiss study (Uebelhart) suggested that 800 mg of chondroitin was nearly as effective as 1200 mg, and that alternating three months on and three months off was just as effective as continuous treatment.

After reviewing all the evidence, including Vangsness' 2009 review of evidence-based medicine for glucosamine and chondroitin in my favorite journal, *Arthroscopy*, I have come down favorably on the side of recommending glucosamine and chondroitin. I have witnessed symptomatic benefits in many patients I have followed.

To round out our discussion of glucosamine and chondroitin, I should add that many formulations of glucosamine and chondroitin come with MSM (methylsulfonylmethane). Many of my patients ask about MSM. The research on MSM is not as compelling as that on glucosamine and chondroitin. Basically, MSM is a good source of sulfur and has a structure similar to DMSO (dimethyl sulfoxide). I mentioned earlier that DMSO is a solvent that aids in the absorption of curcumin. You may not be familiar with DMSO, but years ago it was quite popular among athletes as a salve for joint pain. In the 1970s my mother, who had terrible rheumatoid arthritis, participated in a Yale study on DMSO in rheumatoid patients. I remember its strong garlic odor, which spread throughout our house. (Unfortunately, the DMSO didn't help Mom.)

The studies on MSM have not convinced me to include it on my most-recommended list. However, if it's combined with the glucosamine and chondroitin in the formulation you take, you don't have to worry—it won't hurt you, and there is some favorable research on it.

There is enthusiasm for the combination of glucosamine and chondroitin with other supplements, such as omega-3s (Jerosch 2011) and antioxidants.

RECOMMENDED DAILY DOSAGE	
Glucosamine	1500 mg
Chondroitin	1200 mg

Potential side effects: Does not appear that glucosamine has any effect on blood glucose levels in diabetics. Because glucosamine is made from shellfish shells, and chondroitin can be derived from shark cartilage theoretically they could induce allergic reactions in people with seafood allergy. They can cause soft stools, gas, and a blood-thinning effect. Consult your medical doctor if you are on blood thinners.

LICORICE

When I was a kid, on Friday nights in the summer my mom would make popcorn with butter for when we would watch the Yankees. We were longtime Yankee fans. More often than not, we would also have a bag of licorice, black or red. It's ironic that years later I worked with the Yankees' archrivals, the Boston Red Sox, as an orthopedic consultant, but I never worked with the Yankees. (Starting out life as a Yankee fan and becoming a Red Sox doctor can definitely complicate family dynamics.)

My mom rationalized that the licorice was good for us, because she had heard that it was healthy based on its use in ancient Chinese medicine. What she didn't realize was that red licorice was made of corn syrup, flour, sugar, glycerin, and red dye, and there wasn't any real licorice root in the candy, so it wasn't providing any health benefits. The truth really hurts sometimes.

Licorice *(Glycyrrhiza glabra)* is related to beans and peas, has a pod, and smells of anise. The root of the licorice plant possesses an anti-inflammatory effect. Usually the root is ground up and water is used to extract the active ingredient, glycyrrhizic acid.

Studies have illustrated the anti-inflammatory powers of licorice and its ability to prevent heart disease. Licorice is also an excellent example of how a supplement can reduce inflammation (which helps the joints) and, by doing so, affect many disease processes. For example, diammonium glycyrrhizinate, a licorice derivative, has been shown to lower NFkB activity in colonic mucosa, thereby reducing inflammation in the colonic disease called ulcerative colitis (Yuan 2006).

One must be careful with the dosage of licorice, however. Real licorice can act like aldosterone, a hormone made in the adrenal gland that causes fluid retention, which leads to higher blood pressure. Eating too much "real licorice" can cause dangerously low potassium levels and high blood pressure. It can also have toxic effects on the liver.

Licorice can be very healthy for the cardiovascular system, the colon, and the joints, but it must be monitored closely and should be cycled on and off monthly. I have some concerns about recommending licorice because of the negative blood pressure and potassium side effects, but I have seen it work wonders in some patients, so I am including it here. Because the candy licorice that we buy in the United States isn't an adequate source of the active ingredient and is full of joint-unhealthy sugar, it doesn't have the benefit of real licorice.

My recommendation would be to buy a limited, one-month supply of the supplement so that you can't possibly take it for too long. After taking it for a month, stay off it for a month.

RECOMMENDED DAILY DOSAGE
Licorice extract 1.5 gms (400 mg of glycyrrhizic acid). Take it for no more than one month; then take one month off.
Potential side effects: Can be toxic to the liver; causes low potassium levels and high blood pressure.

N-ACETYL CYSTEINE (NAC)

Free radicals are destructive charged particles that exert their deleterious effects on the cell membrane and DNA. Free radicals play a significant role in aging, as well as producing cytokines, those dastardly molecules, like TNF-alpha, IL-1 beta, and MMPs, which initiate and form the inflammatory cascade. Controlling free radicals is extremely important. For joint health, it is essential to provide as much cysteine as necessary, and you can do this by supplementing with N-acetyl cysteine (NAC). The NAC supplement is processed by the body with glutamate and glycine to form glutathione, the body's most important antioxidant. Glutathione, produced with NAC's help, is then able to scavenge free radicals and protect the body from inflammation. As far back as 1991, scientists in France (Schreck) showed that NAC could counteract H_2O_2 in free radical activation of NFkB. Other supplements also increase glutathione levels, including SAMe, silymarin, and alpha lipoic acid. Each is a reasonable option, but from my experience, NAC is especially effective. Beware that capsules of NAC stink of sulfur—like rotten eggs! You don't have to worry about the smell; keep them in a closed container.

RECOMMENDED DAILY DOSAGE
600 mg
Potential side effects: Can cause stomach upset and diarrhea. NAC is a mild excitotoxin, so it is not good for people with neurologic problems.

MY PATIENT JOHN AND HIS MOTHER-IN-LAW

John came to see me because his back and right hip were bothering him so much that he couldn't play softball up to his expectations. He was thirty-two years old and was a hardworking guy. He was in good shape but was becoming worn down from a laborious job and an intense softball schedule. I placed him on some medication and sent him to physical therapy. He achieved good results with these approaches, but they didn't last. Within months he was back in my office, and soon he missed some work and a number of games due to pain. That's when he became receptive to the thought of adopting a joint-healthy lifestyle. He wanted to discontinue the prescription medicine, and because he didn't have time for regularly scheduled appointments, he wanted to be responsible for his own physical therapy. In addition, he was happy to try to eat better. The problem was that both he and his wife worked long hours, he played a lot of softball, and neither of them cooked. His mother-in-law lived with them and did all the cooking. When I heard about this setup, I bit my tongue, and when he told me he'd simply tell his mother-in-law what to cook, I chuckled to myself, sensing that I hadn't heard the last of this story.

A few weeks went by, and in all honesty, I forgot about John's cooking issue, until one day when I walked into the patient room and there was John, sitting on the exam table, with his mother-in-law in the chair next to him. When I introduced myself to his mother-in-law, John didn't say a word. It was clear that he was petrified. Without any small talk she told me her name, followed by her title, saying, "I'm John's mother-in-law." Without a second's pause she added, "So what am I supposed to cook for him?" What followed was a twenty-minute discussion colored by remarks like:

"Buffalo? You've got to be kidding me. Jane isn't going to go for the thought of someone killing a buffalo."

"No potatoes? What? Are you crazy? John, I don't know what nationality he is, but he's not Irish."

continued

"So, Doctor, you're telling me that he can eat all the eggs he wants. John, I think this doctor is trying to knock you off."

"Organic grass-fed cows? You've got to be kidding me. Doc, do you know how much that costs per pound? Ha, ha, ha! John, he must think you make a lot more money than you do."

Most of the time I didn't know whether to laugh or console John. A week later my assistant slipped me a note.

Doctor D,

Buffalo isn't so bad. I didn't tell Jane it was buffalo. We all like the food.

John is good, and my shoulders and hands feel better, too.

Thanks,

John's mother-in-law

I roared in laughter when I saw that she had actually signed it "John's mother-in-law."

SILYMARIN

Silymarin is extracted from the seeds of milk thistle. University of Texas researchers (Manna 1999) have shown that it inhibits NFkB. Long-known cytoprotective and anti-inflammatory effects of silymarin make it an attractive supplement for a joint-healthy lifestyle. Research conducted by Ashkavand in India in 2012 showed that silymarin was able to reduce the fibrillation of articular cartilage in rats with osteoarthritis. This represents extremely exciting data supporting silymarin as having joint-specific anti-inflammatory value. I started using silymarin more frequently with patients in 2012 and added it to my personal program in 2011. I have started to see some exciting results in patients, and I personally feel it has helped me. Now, with recent experimental data supporting its specific efficacy in helping articular cartilage, I have placed it in my stack of preferred supplements for treating joint pain and inflammation.

As with other supplements, silymarin absorption can be improved by combining it with a phytosome of soy phospholipids. Silymarin–phospholipid complex is sold under the brand name Siliphos.

RECOMMENDED DAILY DOSAGE
200 mg 2 times per day
Potential side effects: Can cause nausea, heartburn, dyspepsia, and transient headache.

SUPPLEMENTS TO WATCH

Sometimes knowing what not to use is just as important as knowing what to use. Always be safe before sorry. The following supplements have been the subject of some promising but conflicting research. I do not currently recommend them, but I may in the future, as more research is conducted. I am including them here because you may hear about them, read about them on the internet, or have a friend recommend them to you. Always proceed with caution before taking supplements that promise magical results without the information and research to back them up. I will keep you abreast of any changes in my recommendations through my website at www.healthyjointsforlife.com.

CITRUS PECTIN

When most of us eat an orange or squeeze a lemon, we throw out the peel. That's too bad, because an important component in the dried peel is citrus pectin. Commercially, it is extracted and used primarily as a gelling agent in jams and jellies. Chemically, it is a polysaccharide, meaning it is a chain of sugars strung together. In this case it is galactose sugars connected end to end. I love what it does for jams and jellies and even jelly beans (I'm guilty of indulging on occasion). I also love what it does to iNOS and COX-2 by inhibiting our foe NFkB. In 2006 Taiwanese researchers (Chen) showed that citrus pectin could modulate iNOS and COX-2 expression in macrophages. It, therefore, could be included in a joint-healthy lifestyle. I know you're not going to start eating orange peels or lemon peels, so citrus pectin will have to come in supplement form, but I want you to know that I am evaluating it presently and will keep you abreast of my results with it through my website at www.healthyjointsforlife.com.

THE JOINT DEVIL, *LIMONCELLO*, AND JOINT HEALTH

My patient Anthony has a strong Italian heritage. He loves going to Arthur Avenue in New York, the famous Italian American area where restaurants and open markets abound. He knows my weakness for dried Italian sausage, and like "the joint devil," he brings me links of inflammation-provoking, but terribly delicious Arthur Avenue dried Italian sausage. I have the darnedest time fighting off the Arthur Avenue dried Italian sausage. If I stick strictly to the joint-healthy diet, an occasional sausage has virtually no symptomatic effect, so I indulge in a couple of slices and love every minute of it. If I ate it every day, I don't think it would be as special, and it would also affect my football-induced knee arthritis.

Recently, Anthony came in to see me, but instead of dried Italian sausage, he brought in sugared lemon rinds. Apparently, after making *limoncello*, the after-dinner Italian liqueur made from lemons, he collects the remnant lemon rinds from the bottom of the barrel, cuts them in thin strips, and rolls them in pure cane sugar. He then eats them as sweet and sour candies or puts them in coffee or espresso as a flavoring.

I suggested that he roll the lemon-rind strips in Truvia instead of cane sugar, and then eating the lemon rinds would give him a joint-healthy dose of citrus pectin without the inflammatory dose of sugar. I haven't convinced my patient Anthony, "the joint devil," to come to our side as of yet, but if he rolls his rinds in Truvia, then I will know he has converted from the dark to the light.

GUGGULSTERONES

I have been very impressed with research investigating the anti-inflammatory properties of guggulsterones, derived from the guggul plant, *Commiphora mukul.* Some have espoused the virtues of gugguls to lower cholesterol and speed up metabolism as a fat burner.

I am excited by studies showing that gugguls inhibit NFkB in synovial cells, pancreatic cells, epithelial cells, and even cancer cells (Lee 2008; Lv 2008; Shishodia 2004). My biggest concern about gugguls is their long-term effects on the thyroid. Studies from the 1980s pointed out that gugguls could stimulate the thyroid (Tripathi 1984). Clinical trials with gugguls have been safe when they have been used for twenty-four weeks and longer. However, there are case reports of thyroid-level changes with gugguls, so monitoring is necessary. I am close to becoming a supporter of gugguls. I am very conservative when it comes to supplements, so the only way I would allow any of my patients to take gugguls is to trial them with physician-followed monitoring of thyroid levels. Once again, I'll keep you abreast of my position on my website at www.healthyjointsforlife.com.

QUERCETIN

Quercetin is found in capers, apples, tea, red onions, red grapes, citrus, tomatoes, broccoli, cherries, raspberries, and cranberries. There is some fascinating research dealing with the ability of quercetin to effect the differentiation of fat cells. A 2008 study by Yang at the University of Georgia determined that the combination of resveratrol and quercetin stopped pre-fat cells from differentiating into fat cells and caused mature fat cells to die (apoptosis). Getting mature fat cells to die is quite an accomplishment, and preventing immature fat cells from becoming mature fat cells is equally impressive. The implications of this for weight loss and weight control are far-reaching, but I haven't seen further research, which has me skeptical.

Quercetin has also been shown to inhibit NFkB and is thought to have beneficial effects on prostate disease, cancer, allergic inflammation, and asthma. I like the effect it has on NFkB and fat cells, especially when combined with resveratrol.

The use of quercetin to magnify the effects of resveratrol has me fascinated. Its effects on fat cells and NFkB make it joint healthy. It's certainly one to watch. I do not have sufficient experience using it with patients yet, so it isn't on my recommended list.

BETAINE

I'd be willing to bet that few people have ever heard of betaine. We eat it in whole wheat, beets, and spinach. Our body can make it from choline. Choline, usually categorized with the B vitamins, is found in egg yolks, soy, wheat germ, and meats. It is part of cell membranes and is also part of the neurotransmitter acetylcholine. Neurotransmitters are the chemical messengers secreted by nerve cells that facilitate the transmission of nerve impulses and muscular contraction.

Betaine's role in maintaining glutathione levels helps with joint health. When glutathione levels wane, free radicals wreak havoc and stimulate NFkB activation. Betaine helps keep NFkB inactive. This was all illustrated quite nicely in a 2007 Korean study by Go in the *Biological & Pharmaceutical Bulletin*.

I recently started to use betaine at home, in my own personal supplement stack, but I haven't used it with more than twenty patients, so I'm not willing to put my stamp of approval on it yet. I have the feeling that it will join my supplement and vitamin recommendations in the near future.

MELATONIN

According to the inflammation theory of aging, free radical production is intimately tied to the process of aging. The theory puts forth that the production of destructive free radicals leads to pathways activating NFkB in the production of inflammatory cytokines. While vitamins A, C, and E are not effective free radical scavengers against aging in metabolic diseases that accompany the aging process, melatonin is. Previously considered only a nighttime sleeping aid, melatonin has been thrust to the forefront by virtue of its antioxidant, and therefore anti-inflammatory potency.

That all sounds good, but there are some serious conflicting reports to consider. There are some concerns about melatonin's effects on the white blood cells known as helper T cells. Melatonin actually increases inflammatory molecule cytokine production in these activated cells (Cutolo 2005; Kalpakcioglu 2009). It was originally thought that the pineal gland was the only producer of melatonin, but it is now known that the white blood cells called lymphocytes produce melatonin in large quantities. If melatonin leads to increased production of cytokines, and if it is produced in larger quantities than originally estimated, then this could be devastating for joint health.

The counterbalancing clinical effect of melatonin on cortisol, secreted by the adrenal glands, is also a concern. Cortisol blocks "bad" prostaglandin production, so the effect of melatonin on cortisol could increase pain. It has been postulated that in situations where there is an insensitivity to cortisol, excessive melatonin production may be the reason.

Anyone who has rheumatoid arthritis, or knows someone who does, realizes that morning stiffness and swelling are significant problems. The nighttime variation in inflammatory molecule cytokines seems to peak at the same time melatonin is highest and cortisol is lowest in the body. In their 2004 paper on the experimental role of melatonin in arthritis, Cardinali et al. explained that melatonin increases cytokine production via its pro-inflammatory effect on the synovial macrophages.

Because of these concerning reports on melatonin, I want to make sure you are aware of melatonin's negative effects on joint health. If you have joint pain and are taking melatonin for sleep, I suggest that you stop the melatonin and see if there is any change in your joint pain.

KAVA

Kava has a fascinating history in the island cultures of the South Pacific. The root of the kava plant is pounded or ground and mixed with water to produce a drink that has a numbing/anesthetic effect on the mouth and an anxiety-relieving effect. Kava is reportedly great for those with social anxiety. Parts of the kava plant can be damaging to the liver, however. Several cases of liver toxicity were reported in 2001, and several countries, including the Netherlands, France, Switzerland, and Canada, have banned kava (U.S. Centers for Disease Control and Prevention 2002).

Kava does inhibit NFkB rather well, its anti-inflammatory effect is notable, and kava at night could be quite relaxing. We've learned the importance of stress reduction on cortisol levels, and you certainly know how much we love to inhibit NFkB. However, the significant side effects of kava are too concerning, so I feel it is important for you to avoid the use of kava.

THE *HEALTHY JOINTS FOR LIFE* SUPPLEMENT STACK

There is no perfect supplement or supplement stack, but this particular stack has performed very well for patients in my practice. Many patients with nonsurgical osteoarthritis have been enrolled in at least three-month trials using the stack. Typically, I include licorice in the first and third month, but not the second, unless the patient has high blood pressure. Previously, in my first study, which featured only omega-3s, I had seen about 58 percent of patients with osteoarthritis improve. I was happy with that, but many other clinical studies from the past have shown that nearly 60 percent of patients get better with a placebo, so I wanted to see if I could do better. My most recent stack upped the ante, with more than 70 percent of patients reporting a notable improvement in symptoms regardless of the severity of their osteoarthritis. And that statistic doesn't really tell the whole story, because many patients using this supplement stack also relay a feeling of well being. Little aches disappear. Energy levels improve, as well. The icing on the cake for many is the change noted in blood cholesterol and triglycerides.

SUPPLEMENT	RECOMMENDED DAILY DOSAGE*
Lutein	10–40 mg 1x/day
Astaxanthin	2–4 mg 1x/day
Vitamin B_6	10–20 mg 1x/day
Vitamin B total mixed	Multi of B_1–B_{12} 1x/day
Vitamin C	500 mg 2x/day
Vitamin D_3	2000–5000 IU 1x/day
Vitamin E total mixed	100 IU 1x/day
Vitamin E gamma-tocotrienol	15 mg 1x/day

continued

SUPPLEMENT	RECOMMENDED DAILY DOSAGE*
Calcium	250 mg 2x/day
Omega-3s	1000 mg 2x/day
PAC/Grape seed extract	200 mg 2x/day
Resveratrol	250 mg 1x/day
Curcumin (biocurcumax)	250–500 mg 2x/day
Boswellia	300 mg 2x/day
Pomegranate extract	250–500 mg 2x/day
Ginger	500–1000 mg 1x/day
Green tea	270 mg total EGCG in 2–3 separate doses
Glucosamine	1500 mg 1x/day
Chondroitin	1200 mg 1x/day
Licorice root (max 1-month cycle)	400 mg of glycyrrhizic acid 1x/day (maximum dose)
NAC	600 mg 1x/day
Silymarin	200 mg 2x/day

* Dosages of proprietary supplements with improved absorption can be lessened

Just like each movie star has his or her detractors, so do the stars of my stack for joint pain. Some cause thinning of the blood, so they are a concern for those on blood thinners, like Plavix or Coumadin. Licorice root can cause high blood pressure and shouldn't be taken for prolonged periods of time. The bioavailability of "regular" curcumin supplements is only a few hours. But their benefits, when they are taken at the appropriate dosage and with an awareness of potential side effects, can far outweigh their risks.

I'm sure you're wondering why I didn't include quercetin, guggulsterones, betaine, citrus pectin, kava, and melatonin in my stack, especially because there is enticing research substantiating their benefits. The answers are quite simple. I'm concerned about the possible side effects of kava and melatonin, so I'm not willing to give them a recommendation. But I want you to know about them in case someone recommends them to you. Knowing what not to take can be very valuable. I'm concerned about the reports of joint pain associated with quercetin and want to see more studies and information before giving a full-fledged recommendation. I have started using guggulsterones on select patients, but I am still worried about possible negative thyroid effect with prolonged use. Because I'm worried about the side effects, I won't give my recommendation until I closely follow a larger number of patients. I must admit, though, that guggulsterones do look promising, and since I haven't seen thyroid side effects, I am getting closer to a recommendation. The others, citrus pectin and betaine, are also alluring, but I don't have enough positive experience with them at this time to make a surefire recommendation. I will be using them with appropriate patients soon and will be able to pass this information on in future writings on my website at www.healthyjointsforlife.com.

REAL PEOPLE, REAL RESULTS

"After I developed serious stomach problems taking NSAIDs, Dr. Diana placed me on his supplement stack, and at first I thought it was crazy. I was taking dozens of pills daily. And I'm not into taking pills in the first place. After a couple of weeks I was convinced I was crazy, because I didn't feel a thing. I almost gave up. Dr. Diana told me to be patient, something I'm not really good at. By the end of eight weeks I was the most-surprised guy in town. I felt better, noticeably better. Now I think it's crazy not to take the stack!"

"I went to Dr. Diana, as directed by my medical doctor, for my sports-induced knee pain, expecting a recommendation for surgery. After all, he is a surgeon! Instead, I came out of

continued

the office with a list of supplements. The list sat on my desk until my wife convinced me to start on the supplements, and I also started eating differently, and within a week I felt different. When I revisited the doc, he downplayed the initial results! He told me that my initial results might be just wishful thinking. After twelve weeks he beamed with pride and shook my hand. The results were no longer wishful, but the real thing."

"The doc gave me a bunch of supplements to take, and my joint pain improved. I was happy. And then I went to my cardiologist to get my cholesterol checked, and the supplements, including the omega-3s, must have reduced my cholesterol, too! My cardiologist was even happier!"

"I have really bad osteoarthritis. Conventional treatments from my medical doctor weren't helping me, so I went to the orthopedic surgeon Dr. Diana. I have a bunch of medical problems, so Dr. Diana told me to try some omega-3s and a dozen other supplements. After a while I felt quite a bit better, but I still had some pain, so he restarted me on an NSAID and that was just what I needed. The combination of supplements and mainstream NSAIDs did it. Who would have thought a surgeon would be giving me supplements and then combining them with mainstream meds? I'm thankful."

Throughout the eight-week program (Chapters 6 to 14) I will explain how to add these supplements to your daily diet. As I have noted in this chapter, there is compelling scientific research that supports including these supplements in your new joint-healthy lifestyle. Supplements can be pricey, but the program groups them into four levels and allows you to choose what level of supplements you'd like to take. Supplements can be found in health-food stores, chain stores like GNC, CVS, and Wal-Mart, and online. Visit www.healthyjointsforlife.com for a list of options and simplified shopping.

CHAPTER 5

MOVE:
How Exercise Helps You
Move Better and Feel Better

EXERCISE HELPS YOUR JOINTS ON MOLECULAR, METABOLIC, AND mechanical levels. But when you suffer from joint pain, the idea of exercising can be daunting. There is a fine line between exercising enough to keep your joints flexible, strong, and healthy and exercising too much, which can lead to an increase in pain or joint damage. I will help you find the balance. My exercise program is based on choosing exercises that are best suited to your degree of joint pain. Those of you with less pain can exercise more frequently and with more intensity. Those of you with more pain can exercise enough to get the benefits, without causing further pain.

On a molecular basis, exercise benefits joints by stimulating the production of cartilage matrix and synovial fluid. The metabolic effects of exercise inhibit NFkB and modulate insulin. On a mechanical basis, muscles, tendons, ligaments, and bones are strengthened by exercise. Weight loss, achieved through exercise, decreases stress on the joints. The psychological advantages are vast.

A successful exercise program needs to be tailored to your needs. Any program that is painful or uninspiring, or that does not provide a challenge, is doomed to fail. This may seem obvious, but if you are bored or in pain, you will not want to exercise. Adding music, TV, fresh air, or different scenery, or varying your workouts, can keep you motivated. If you are bored, you will become more aware of your pain and it will stop you in your tracks.

It is sometimes difficult to differentiate between the pain that means you should stop and the pain that is associated with fatigue and/or osteoarthritis. It's important to know that you can disregard and battle through some pains. Learning the difference between pain related to injury, as opposed to soreness, comes with experience. If the pain does not lead to swelling and subsequent prolonged, increased pain, then you can and should battle through it. If the pain is followed by swelling and significantly increased pain the following day, then you need to revise your program.

Your exercise plan needs to be performed regularly, a total of roughly two and a half to three and a half hours per week, and should include aerobic exercise, resistance training (weights or resistance bands), and flexibility training. It is important that you make the time to exercise—your joints will thank you!

CHOOSING EXERCISES WISELY

Remember, the type and intensity of the exercise you choose should be based on the severity of your joint disease and your general health status. Please be sure to consult with your doctor before embarking on an exercise program.

A TALE OF TWO PATIENTS

In my practice I see patients who are as different from one another as night and day. While they may seek my advice and expertise because they have joint pain, the search for the solutions to their problems is often as individual as they are. However, at the core of helping them is finding a balance between exercising enough so that their joints are strengthened but not so much that they are damaged due to overuse. Sometimes finding the balance can be challenging, as you'll see from the following patients.

Marguerite, a forty-five-year-old marathon runner, has managed to run her joints and heart into near ruin. Her knees are 50 percent worn-out, and her heart is in and out of rhythm. During the years I have been her orthopedic sports medicine surgeon, she has demoralized and dismissed several cardiologists. It makes me wonder when and if she'll fire me. Most recently, I've spent less of my time diagnosing and treating her knees than I have begging her to vary and decrease her workouts. Marguerite is addicted to running, to the point where she ignores her pain to soothe her psyche. Many runners chase the runner's high—an endorphin surge produced by the brain. Marguerite, like many who run, will do so at any cost, including self-destruction. I've done everything I can to help her knees, realizing that the better I make her feel, the more she runs and the worse her overall health becomes. After our appointments I leave her room convinced I've made her knees better for the short term but concerned her running will lead to further problems.

The contrast between Marguerite and James, a fifty-eight-year-old former football player, is glaring, and especially perplexing. I'm convinced that James logs more hours

continued

on a couch than anyone short of a furniture salesperson. The only running he does is to the store to buy more pretzels and beer. He loves pizza. He has it delivered to minimize his inconvenience and goes so far as to season it with extra salt. I admire his honesty when he admits his joint-related sins.

Naturally, James is overweight and, as bad fortune would have it, works as a plumber, and so he must kneel for extended periods of time. I'd estimate that over a decade I've seen him twenty-five times for knee pain. At each office visit we discuss his rather mild knee problem, which is symptomatic because he eats tremendous quantities of, well, junk and refuses to exercise. A night watching *Monday Night Football* with a double bacon cheeseburger, nachos, fries, and a few wings is his idea of healthy eating. On his worst nights I'm convinced he simply eats trans fats and washes them down with high fructose corn syrup.

Believe it or not, at times James has achieved amazing results from weight reduction, healthy eating, and mild but consistent exercise. But his joint health doesn't last for long. James specializes in repeated relapses. One time he and his buddy decided they would enter a tag team eating competition. Their training schedule was intense and he gained thirty-five pounds, which, of course, led to his knees swelling. Another time he sprained an ankle while carrying a washing machine down a client's stairwell. For some reason, he wore clogs to work that day. As a result of the sprain, he didn't exercise for two months and ate as badly as ever. You guessed correctly: he landed back in my office with knee pain—again.

After evaluating Marguerite, my marathon runner, and then James, my favorite couch potato plumber, I had seemingly traveled through the clinical twilight zone and seen the gamut of excesses. These two perfectly wonderful and extreme patients have provided undeniable clinical evidence for the importance of an appropriate exercise program. And an appropriate exercise program is what I want you to adopt to keep your joints healthy and mobile. Armed with the knowledge of what happens with the extremes of exercise, we can better understand what exercise does to our joints both on a mechanical (physical) level and on the molecular level.

THE MECHANICAL EFFECT OF EXERCISE

Over the last two decades many research centers have documented how motion with the intermittent compression of cartilage—supplied by the right kind of exercise, like walking—leads to the production of healthy extracellular matrix. Constant static compression, like constant kneeling, has been shown to degrade matrix (Kim 2012). Taking a daily walk is part of a joint-healthy lifestyle, whereas kneeling all day long, installing carpeting, is not.

As a medical student, I learned from doctors at Newington Children's Hospital in Connecticut that joint motion stimulates the healthy production of synovial fluid, while immobilization does the opposite (Salter 1989). The reason a patient will experience stiffness after being in a cast is in part due to the lack of synovial fluid production during the time the joint was immobilized. Synovial fluid helps nourish the articular cartilage and promotes near frictionless motion. Ordinary motion via light exercise, household chores, or activities of daily living is joint healthy. Being a total couch potato is anything but joint healthy.

During the excruciatingly hot August football practices in Miami, we half joked that if practice didn't kill you, it only made you stronger.

Science shows that there is some truth to that thought, the caveat being that a tissue that is stressed appropriately will strengthen. Too much stress will cause problems, but the *right amount* of stress is helpful. Muscles, tendons, ligaments, and bones are no exceptions to that rule, each showing improved strength in response to the stress of an appropriate level of exercise.

THE IMPORTANCE OF MUSCLE STRENGTH

One of the most obvious benefits of exercise is maintaining or improving muscle strength. Improved muscle strength also benefits the joints. Because muscles move joints, strong muscles allow for improved joint tracking. For example, the kneecap will not travel in its groove appropriately unless the thigh muscles support and guide it. If the muscles don't guide the kneecap symmetrically, then the ligaments on one side or the other will be overloaded. In this scenario, the strain of regular use leads to ligament pain in the short term and joint cartilage wear over time. If the muscles around the kneecap allow the kneecap to tilt in its track inappropriately, then one side of the kneecap will absorb most of the stress, leading to excess wear on that side. The following two diagrams illustrate what I'm saying quite nicely.

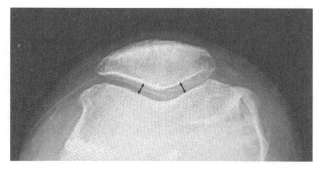

Even stress distribution

Arthritic Spur

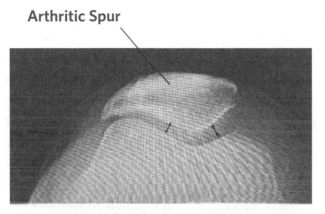

Uneven stress distribution leading to arthritis

Muscles also reduce joint stress by absorbing forces before they can impact and damage the joint. If you were to jump off a three-foot wall and land on your feet with your knees fully extended, or "straight," your knees would feel an incredible jolt. If you were to land on your feet with your knees bent, your thigh muscles would absorb the majority of the force and a manageable amount of stress would be felt by your knee joints.

Muscle strength also positively impacts coordination and safety. One of the largest causes of pain, suffering, and death in the elderly is hip fracture. Statistics show that more than 50 percent of elderly persons with hip fractures die within one year. The hip fracture leads to a cascade of problems, including inactivity, that are associated with significant mortality rates. Decrease falls by improving strength and coordination and you've reduced one of the most common causes of premature death in the elderly.

The ligaments around the joint are the first line of defense against trauma, because they provide constant support around the joint. Since they are always engaged, ligaments provide instantaneous protection. Muscles also protect the joint but must be contracted to provide protection. The time it takes to contract makes the muscles an important but secondary line of defense. If you slip on ice and feel your knee beginning to pull the wrong way, healthy ligaments will prevent the knee from going out of place and then the muscles will be activated, too. Moderate joint stress via exercise strengthens the collagen cross-links in ligaments, leading to a better-stabilized joint. Stronger ligaments do not tear easily and protect the joint surfaces from damage (Uzel 2011). Exercises that stress and strengthen the ligaments are an essential part of the *Healthy Joints for Life* exercise program.

EXERCISE AND YOUR BONES

The force of weight-bearing exercise—climbing stairs, walking, or playing tennis, to name a few—stimulates the bone to gain strength and density. Exercise is essential to bone health and strength. As we age, bone density can decrease, making weight-bearing exercise all the more important. Less dense bones are more prone to becoming brittle and can break more easily. The age-related weakening of bones (osteoporosis) can be countered by weight-bearing exercise. It is important to maintain bone strength as you age, because what would be a simple fall for a teenager, who jumps right back up, can cause a broken hip or wrist in a person with osteoporosis. Strong bones keep you from sustaining bone damage from slips or falls.

Additionally, the articular cartilage that protects the ends of your bones cannot be healthy if the underlying, supporting bone is not strong. Consider what might happen to you and your tiled kitchen floor if the plywood subfloor were missing. When you stepped on the floor, you would crack the tile, fall through the floor, and land in the basement. Similarly, without the underlying strong bone, the articular cartilage would bend, fissure, and degenerate.

Cyclic loading exercise—moving and bearing weight, like when biking, walking, and running, where you do a cycle, step, or revolution and repeat it over and over—provides molecular stimulus for the production of cartilage matrix. Motion also stimulates the production of lubricating synovial fluid.

EXERCISE, WEIGHT LOSS, INSULIN, AND NFkB

For the purpose of joint-pain relief, weight loss lessens the overall mechanical load on the joints, but keeping weight under control can also have a molecular effect on inflammation. In 2009 Carlsen et al. from Oslo, Norway, showed that obesity leads to an increased baseline level of NFkB activity and, therefore, inflammation. Two years earlier other investigators found similar effects on NFkB in obese patients. Researchers also discovered that exercise generates increased glutathione—the body's most powerful antioxidant. The more antioxidants, the better, as anything that fights free radicals is ultimately fighting NFkB and its partner in crime, inflammation. In their 2007 paper on human adipose tissue (fat) Clement and Langin note, "The identification of a moderate increase in circulating inflammatory factors in obese subjects are observations contributing to the concept that human obesity is a chronic inflammatory illness." This tells us that even without the mechanical considerations of joint stress, obesity is painful to joints, simply because it's inflammatory.

Another by-product of being trim is keeping your cells sensitive to insulin. If your cells are not sensitive to insulin, then more insulin is necessary to maintain normal levels of glucose. Imagine two people, one with insulin resistance and the other with normal sensitivity to insulin. The person with insulin resistance might need to secrete twice as much insulin to keep their blood glucose levels normal, but at the same time the greater levels of insulin bathe all cells and increase NFkB. Heightened inflammation results. In contradistinction, the person with normal insulin sensitivity has half as much circulating insulin and, therefore, less inflammation. In addition, the higher the level of insulin is in your body, the more your fatty acid synthetase and HMG-CoA reductase enzymes will be triggered for insulin-related fat production and cholesterol production. Exercise will certainly burn calories, but it will also decrease insulin levels, which will decrease fat- and cholesterol-producing enzymes.

Muscle, tendons, ligaments, and bone are strengthened by exercise. NFkB and insulin are both controlled at a molecular level. You've always been told that exercise is good for you, but now you know why, right down to the molecular level.

GETTING MOTIVATED TO EXERCISE

Perhaps the biggest hurdle concerning exercise is getting people to *do* any! Yes, *any!* For decades I have been recommending that my patients exercise. When I was a young doctor, it didn't take me long to realize that recommendations alone are rarely enough. You have to find the key that unlocks a person's inner motivation. I've had to develop a litany of techniques to try to find the key to motivate people to exercise. I've found that each tactic that I've employed has had some wins and some losses.

Motivational talks will often work. Recently, I had great success with a patient and old teammate who was having terrible joint pain. He was starting to feel the effects of age, arthritis, and weight gain. After talking to him about the old days and reliving some of our past victories, he became motivated to rekindle the past with an exercise program. In six months he lost thirty burdensome pounds and the majority of his joint pain. His own words tell the end result best. "I haven't felt this good in twenty years."

I have another patient who responded especially well to thoughts of the years before she had her children. She and her husband enjoyed many vacations to the island of Aruba. When I mentioned that my wife and I were considering a trip there, she promised to bring pictures of her vacations to her next appointment. One of those pictures showed her dancing with her husband in front of a five-piece steel band, with her hair blowing, her hips swiveling, and a smile reaching from ear to ear. It was an absolutely amazing picture, capturing the spirit and joy of the moment. She wanted that moment back and was willing to work for it. Within three months she had lost twenty-four pounds, and her legs felt good enough to dance again.

Many of my patients enjoy reminiscing, and pictures from the past can be great motivators. That bathing suit shot from ten years ago juxtaposed with a more recent, and perhaps unflattering, photo can appeal to the vanity in all of us. Glancing at those pictures after taping them to the refrigerator or pantry door can be a vivid reminder of a goal. I absolutely love the idea of a photo shoot. I think it is an incredible idea to schedule a photo shoot with a photographer for three months from when you start my program to inject some additional motivation and discipline into your program. Having the photo shoot on your calendar keeps the end goal in mind. Frankly, it's a lot cheaper to have a photo shoot than to continue buying pain medicines or paying for failed diet plans. If you have the photo shoot, send the before and after pictures to www.healthyjointsforlife.com. We'd love to show off your success.

For some, motivation comes in the form of a goal, but with a slight twist. For these patients the goal is less about how great they will feel (less joint pain) and more about a reward they promise themselves when they reach a goal weight or get working out consistently. A new sultry dress, a vacation to Italy, or a day at the local spa are a few of the rewards I've seen that entice patients into the gym.

My brother is the ultimate example of a competition-oriented exerciser. He needs a competition to ensure that he doesn't skip exercising. There must be a reward at the end for the winner, no matter how insignificant, even if it's nothing more than bragging rights. On one occasion my brother lost thirty-two pounds with gentle exercise. For him competition is the key. And it doesn't really matter with whom he is competing—he'll take on a challenge with a friend, coworker, his wife, or even me!

For some people, fear is a great motivator. A talk stressing the downhill spiral of inactivity, obesity, joint disease, and heart disease, and the subsequent need for joint replacement and heart surgery, can be powerful. I have been known to show graphic images of knee replacement surgery to kick-start a patient's exercise program. I won't subject you to these photos, but keep in mind that surgery is no fun, and if you can stave off the deterioration of your joints that comes with inactivity, you will be better off.

For many of my patients, from Yale professors to steelworkers to stay-at-home moms and dads, simple reasoning works best. I explain the scientific basis for exercise, and once they understand what's at stake and, more important, what they can do about it, they are committed to getting moving.

One of my favorite patients, a forty-one-year-old mother of two young boys, failed to respond to my best motivational talks. I asked her to do it for her husband and children. It didn't work. Pictures from years past didn't work; reminiscing didn't, either. Rewards didn't entice her in the least. She didn't have a competitive bone in her body, so competition, my brother's favorite motivation, didn't do anything for her. I showed her the photos of replacement surgery, but she looked at them fearlessly. I saw my opening when she showed a surprising academic interest in the gory surgical photos. It turns out that she was a biology major in college, and when I explained the science of matrix synthesis, she ate it up. When she learned about what exercise was doing to her joints on a cellular level, it sparked her interest to the point where she told her husband and kids all about it over dinner that night. She started an exercise program the next day. I never would have guessed that my explaining the science behind the exercise would be the key to getting her moving, but I try not to argue with success.

I never know what is going to work on a patient. Here are some examples of my old tricks that I've used to get patients ready to exercise. I am confident that you really want to do everything possible to help your joints. Dig deep and find the key that will motivate you. I know you want to reduce your pain. Think of all the wonderful things that life has to offer when your pain is under control.

- **Being able to play with your kids/grandkids.** Be a better parent by being less grouchy and more available and willing to be active.
- **Enjoy being active** with your spouse.
- **A social event where you want to look your best?** Enjoy cocktail parties, where you are forced to stand.
- **A high school or college reunion?** Look better and feel more vital.
- **Enjoy a reward that is special to you**—a day at the spa, a trip to a museum, a vacation.
- **Being able to participate in a sport that you love,** such as tennis, golf, running, and so on.
- **Engage in daily activities**—housework, commuting to work, gardening, walking the dog—with no pain.
- **Shop without pain.**
- **Work without having to ice down** when you get home.
- **Walk without a limp,** never having to answer that repetitive and irritating question, "Why are you limping?"
- **Sit in a restaurant booth** and a theater, cinema, airplane, or stadium seat without experiencing that crippling stiffness upon rising.

- **Enjoy your home fully** by going up and down stairs without pain. (I dreaded carrying the kids up the stairs to bed when they were little. Now, I can do it easily.)
- **Enjoy rock climbing,** nature hikes, or kayaking. You can't get in a kayak if you can't bend well.

HOW TO EXERCISE FOR JOINT-PAIN RELIEF

People avoid exercise when it hurts. I'm assuming that is why you may not be moving as much as would be good for you. That's why it is so important to avoid your personal pain threshold that leads you to stop exercising. We all have a point of no return. If I do an incredibly rigorous workout that really burns my muscles and gets me out of breath, I tend to avoid exercising the next day. Part of my brain congratulates me on completing a great workout, while another part begs not to do it again. There was just too much pain. For me, and most others, pain trumps everything else. Exercise programs, therefore, need to be challenging, but not to the point of "I'll never do that again." A little muscle soreness, especially when you are doing something new, is to be expected, but not so much that you don't want to exercise again or can't due to pain. I'm sure you've heard the expression "No pain, no gain." Well, my motto (and you can feel free to adopt it as your own) is a little different, "Too much pain and there will be no gain." Exercise needs to be pleasant and engaging. You have to be willing to do it consistently, and with some effort, in order to make progress.

You don't have to absolutely love your workout, but the type of exercise you choose needs to be interesting and fun. For many, boredom is a huge obstacle to maintaining an exercise program. I'm convinced that boredom can also lower your pain threshold. If you're running or walking on a treadmill in the gym *without* listening to music or watching an interesting TV program, the only thing you will be able to think about is how your knees hurt, how you hate to sweat, how you're out of breath, and how you have too much time left on your workout timer. If you find that by exercising on your own, you won't put in the effort or keep at it, try a class where you are getting instruction from the teacher and inspiration from your classmates. Boredom forces you to concentrate on the pain, exposing and magnifying it. Boredom is an exercise killer.

After two decades of seeing patients, I know that many of you don't like exercise or are not interested in exercising. But I also know that there is irrefutable evidence that exercising can help you feel less pain. I won't ask you to go out and train for a marathon or hit the gym every day for hours. I want you to discover ways to exercise that make you feel good and that help your joints but also give you a sense of accomplishment. A walk around the block on a beautiful day can be just what the doctor ordered.

YOUR EXERCISE PROGRAM

Before you embark on an exercise program, you will need to really think about what you are going to do. In order to create your road map to exercise success, you need to make decisions about:

- When you will exercise
- Where you will exercise
- What type of exercise you will do, being sure to include these three essential components:
    - Aerobic exercise
    - Resistance training
    - Flexibility training

- Whether or not you need to seek professional guidance in developing your exercise plan. This could mean working with your doctor or a personal trainer, or seeking information from the staff at your gym.

Not having enough time is a big excuse for many of my patients, and I'm sure the excuse that you don't have time for exercise has occurred to you, as well. Notice how I didn't mince words. I said, *"Excuse."* Don Shula, my coach when I played for the Miami Dolphins, didn't want excuses. Offer an excuse, and he would verbally undress you in front of the whole team. Mental errors were not tolerated, and excuses were, well, inexcusable. Nobody offered him an excuse more than once. There was a quick learning curve. With excuses came a ticket out the door.

My friend and fellow running back, Larry Cowan, was drafted out of Jackson State by the Dolphins in the seventh round in 1982, the same year I was drafted in the fifth round. Larry had a great preseason camp, and the media was touting him as the next Mercury Morris. Some of you may remember Mercury as an electrifying running back from the Dolphins' Super Bowl VII and VIII championship teams, where he teamed up with other Dolphin running backs you might be familiar with, Jim Kiick and Larry Csonka. As a kid, I loved the way that Mercury played, and I could see Larry's immense talent, as well. Larry Cowan had great speed, like Mercury, and was being given the chance to run back kickoffs when he started to fumble the ball. Coach Shula didn't like fumbling. Larry fumbled a couple of times and within days was released and picked up by the New England Patriots. In Coach Shula's mind there was no excuse for fumbling. Coach Shula sent a clear message to our team, which each of us clearly understood. Seeing my friend and teammate leave troubled me, more than you might imagine. However, through that experience I learned a valuable lesson that I would never forget. You can learn from Larry's misfortune, as well. Just like there was no excuse for fumbling, there are many things in life for which there can be no excuse. There is no excuse for not exercising.

Make room in your schedule for twenty-minute to one-hour exercise sessions at least three times a week. You can certainly do more, but in most cases you need to do only twenty minutes of exercise, plus a short warm-up period, to get results. Remember, more is not always better. If you push too hard, you increase the risk of suffering an overuse injury.

IF YOU OVERDO

If pain or swelling occurs as a result of exercise, there are a couple of things you can do to calm the inflammation and reduce the pain. An easy way to remember the solution is the acronym RICE: Rest, Ice, Compression, and Elevation. So take a break, get some ice on that joint (twenty minutes on and ten minutes off for one hour), use some light pressure to keep the ice directly on the joint but not directly on the skin, and keep the joint elevated above your heart (particularly important for swelling in your lower extremities).

The time of day when you exercise isn't as important as simply getting some exercise into your day. Do it when you get up, at lunch, right after work, or before bed. It's up to you. Maybe you can use an exercise bike in your bedroom or a treadmill at your local gym, or bring a pair of sneakers with you to work for a walk during your lunchtime break. At a minimum, squeeze mildly strenuous exercise into your busy schedule. Preferably, do twenty minutes of moderate aerobic exercise, meaning exercise that elevates your heart rate to a specific percentage of its maximum rate (see page 158 for information on calculating your maximum heart rate). I know Coach Shula didn't tolerate hearing any type of excuse. He used to say, "Excuses are for losing players and teams." To say that you don't have twenty measly minutes to work exercise into your schedule is just an excuse. On the rare occasions when my kids get in trouble, my wife will say, "Wait till Dad hears about this." While that scares my kids, I don't think you'll find that idea quite as threatening. I'm a disciplining Dad, not a disciplining doctor, but I do know a man who scared the heck out of me, Coach Don Shula. He made a living out of teaching discipline to men who were already darned disciplined. I'm not going to say he's going to come after you, but I will say this: If you don't exercise, the person in your life, whether it's your wife, husband, or workout partner, is going to know. That should provide some motivation. And, even more important, you are going to know because your joints will continue to hurt. Consider yourself warned. In my situation it's been thirty years and I still wouldn't want Coach Shula to hear that I missed a workout. I never missed a workout as a Miami Dolphin, but I do remember missing a block on one occasion. While attempting to make that block, I ducked my head and completely missed my target. My teammate got crunched. Coach made sure that I would not make that mistake again. In a flurry of quite descriptive single-syllable words, "#$%&@*," Coach Shula explained to me that he didn't like my technique. I never ducked my head again.

Where you choose to exercise will, in fact, be related to what your time availability is. If you have only a twenty-minute block of time, you won't have time to drive to a gym. You will need to exercise at home or perhaps do something while you are at work. I encourage you to spend the time adjusting your schedule to put in exercise sessions. Make those sessions definite appointments in your date book, calendar, or smartphone. If you are pressed for time, don't be too hard on yourself, especially at first. Remember, if you can exercise for only eight minutes, that's better than doing nothing for eight minutes. Be flexible concerning where you exercise, when you exercise, and what type of exercises you're willing to do. Don't let the thought of exercising become overwhelming. You need a time-efficient and enjoyable exercise program. Inflexibility, or thinking that you have to devote hours of time, becomes the ultimate excuse. When I hear from patients that they don't have the time to exercise, I tell them that is just an excuse. Just like Coach Shula, I don't like or accept excuses. Make an honest effort and your joints will feel much better.

The exercise program that you adopt needs to incorporate aerobic activities, which will burn calories, decrease general inflammation levels, keep your cells sensitive to insulin, move your joints without overload, and, as a bonus, maintain a healthy heart. Our joints love a lighter load, so keeping your weight down is important. Moderate exercise will strengthen bones and ligaments and will foster healthy joint lubrication.

AEROBIC EXERCISE

Aerobic exercise is at the core of a good exercise plan. The good news is that there are many ways to exercise aerobically. Some of you will be quite familiar with the term, but others might not. Basically, aerobic exercise is any exercise of prolonged moderate intensity, like stationary biking or walking. The body uses two different pathways to provide energy for muscles during movement. One utilizes oxygen (aerobic) and the other doesn't (anaerobic). Muscles can work without oxygen over a short period of time, *anaerobic* exercise, but ultimately, prolonged exercise needs to be done aerobically, with oxygen. Sprinting is an example of anaerobic exercise. You could probably hold your breath and sprint forty yards. You couldn't do that for the mile run!

Exercises like jogging/running, biking, rowing, elliptical training, and swimming are aerobic. Any activity that raises your baseline heart rate to 60 to 70 percent of your *maximum heart rate* (see below) over an extended period of time is going to be aerobic. You could sprint for thirty seconds and get your heart rate to 60 to 70 percent, but that's anaerobic; for aerobic exercise, you have to maintain that heart rate for enough time so that the cells have to use energy via aerobic pathways. Exercise videos or calisthenics can do the job. Spinning classes are great. Walking at a brisk rate is fine. You can jump rope. The possibilities are varied, and the good news is that you get to choose which one you like to do best.

It's easy to calculate your maximum heart rate: 220 – your age = maximum heart rate. To calculate your target heart rate (60 to 70 percent of your maximum heart rate), multiply your maximum heart rate by .60 for the low end and .70 for the high end. For example, if you are fifty years old, your maximum heart rate is 170 (220 – 50). Your target heart rate of 60 to 70 percent of your maximum heart rate is 102 to 119 beats per minute (170 x .6 = 102; 170 x .7 = 119). If you can maintain that heart rate for twenty to thirty minutes, three to four times per week, you are hitting the sweet spot. The following table will give you a rough estimate of age and target heart rate.

The easiest way to measure your heartbeats per minute is to put your index finger on the pulse of your opposite wrist. This is located on the thumb side of the wrist, at the base of your palm. Feel around for the pulsating artery, and don't worry if you don't feel it at first. It can be hard to find if you haven't done it before. Keep feeling with varying degrees of pressure and you'll find it. Count the pulses in fifteen seconds and multiply by four to get your heartbeats per minute.

AGE	TARGET HEART RATE (beats per minute)
30	114–133
40	108–126
50	102–119
60	96–112
70	90–105
80	84–98

If you aren't into numbers and monitoring your pulse rate as you exercise, some say that a good way to judge your effort is to take the talk test: you should be able to talk but not sing when you've hit the moderate exercise level.

WARNING! BETA-BLOCKERS AND HEART RATE

Many patients with high blood pressure or heart problems are on medications called beta-blockers—Inderal, Tenormin, Lopressor, Toprol-XL, and Coreg, among others. These medications block specific receptors, called beta-receptors, that help to control heart rate. Patients on beta-blockers may have heart rates controlled to the point where they may not be able to raise their heart rates to the levels that I have recommended for appropriate exercise. Trying to attain recommended heart rates may be dangerous if you are on beta-blockers, so please consult your cardiologist if you are on beta-blockers before engaging in exercise, and seek his or her advice on the proper level of exercise for you and your health.

Choosing the right exercise may mean the difference between joints that swell and hurt and joints that feel better. The length and intensity of exercise will also be especially important. The most common form of aerobic exercise is *steady-rate training,* where you maintain your speed and effort consistently during the time you are, for example, running or biking. While there is nothing wrong with steady-rate training, I recommend a technique called *interval training,* because it adds variety to your workout and challenges you, potentially staving off boredom. Interval training has also been shown to burn calories and raise metabolic rate better than steady-rate aerobic activity (Burke 1994). In an interval training program a lower level of intensity will be maintained for about three minutes, followed by one minute of higher-intensity exercise. This is referred to as a 3:1 ratio. A twenty-minute workout would consist of five cycles of three minutes of low-intensity activity and one minute of higher intensity. You can use heart rate to determine lower intensity, perhaps 60 percent of maximum heart rate (about 100 beats per minute for a fifty-year-old), and to determine higher intensity, perhaps 75 percent of maximum heart rate (about 130 beats per minute for a fifty-year-old).

Interval training can be done while pedaling on a spin bike or running on a treadmill. You can do it while jumping rope or walking or doing calisthenics (jumping jacks, sit-ups, and so on), simply by varying the intensity. How you accomplish elevating your heart rate is up to you. Always be sure it isn't too difficult, and to keep it from being boring, exercise with a friend or a group, listen to music, watch TV, or enjoy the beautiful scenery on a country road.

Keep in mind that there is a big difference between exercising for health and exercising for maximizing performance. If I'm training an athlete for performance, I'll introduce sports-specific high-intensity interval training. For the purposes of joint health, you don't need to train to be an Olympian, but you can still use the science of sports medicine to help you train smarter, for better results—including weight loss.

An amazing study by Tremblay in 1994 compared interval training with steady-rate training. The mind-boggling result was that interval training led to greater fat loss than steady-rate training, even though the number of calories burned by the interval training was 50 percent less than that of the steady-rate exercise. The interval training consumed less time, burned fewer calories, yet led to more fat loss! This doesn't seem logical, but this result can be explained by some fancy metabolic footwork. Muscle enzyme systems for fat metabolism get revved up by interval training. As those enzyme systems rev up, they can better utilize fat instead of carbohydrates for energy. This is a prime example of how it is better to exercise efficiently than extensively. As is always the case, exercising smart trumps exercising with brute force. (If you prefer steady-rate training, fat burning is felt to occur at approximately 65 percent of maximum heart rate, right smack in the middle of the target zone I've recommended.)

Those with more severe arthritis need special consideration. If your joint pains are in your upper extremities, you don't have to worry about the following bit of information, but if you have lower-extremity pain, then the following rules pertain to you. Weight-bearing exercises, like walking and running, are more stressful than gentler, less ballistic exercises, like elliptical training or step/stair training. Non-weight-bearing exercises, like rowing and biking, where the equipment supports your weight, are less stressful on your joints than walking, running, step/stair training, and elliptical training. Swimming is the ultimate exercise for people with joint complaints. Nothing is easier on the joints than swimming, because the water buoys the joints in ways that air cannot. If you happen to be a water person, I encourage you to take advantage of water's wonderful benefits for your joints. My only caveat about swimming is to remember that weight-bearing exercise strengthen bones. For those who can tolerate weight-bearing exercise, it plays a very important role in preventing osteoporosis. If your joint pain won't allow you to engage in weight-bearing exercise, then do the exercises you can tolerate and know that you are doing appropriate exercise for your unique health situation. As your pain decreases, you may find that you are able to add a mild weight-bearing exercise, like walking, to your workouts.

Many people enjoy the entertainment and motivation supplied by exercise videos. They can be really fun and incredibly effective. Realize, however, that exercise videos can be high or low impact. For example, a step workout might put more strain on your joints than a Pilates or yoga workout. If your favorite video has you bouncing up and down, then it is high impact and you need to be careful. Joint pain may be only hours away. Be very careful of the activity you choose, because for people with joint arthritis, there is a very thin line between beneficial exercise and damaging exercise.

A close friend who is also a foot and ankle surgeon in my practice was approaching his fiftieth birthday and decided it was time to get into great shape. He was excited and was going to do a program with his son, a budding high school athlete. He told me he had decided on an exercise program primarily featuring CrossFit, which is a competitive high-intensity aerobic and resistance-training fitness program. My friend had some concerns about exercising, because he had reconstructive surgery on one of his knees many years earlier, but he wasn't having too much pain. He had been a high school athlete and was confident that he could do it. For some people (like his son), this type of a program can be perfect. For people with arthritic joints, however, this type of a program can be trouble. I expressed my strong reservations because of his knee and because I see so many middle-aged weekend warriors hurt themselves in high-intensity exercise programs, even if they don't have arthritis. Despite my admonitions, he dove right in. What he learned is that athletes who are training for competition are the ones who should be engaging in this type of intense training. Within two months he was injured, limping at work, and complaining of significant knee pain. Naturally, I helped him, and he is now doing fine. These types of problems can be avoided. Even if you are or were athletic, remember, exercising smart trumps exercising with brute force.

I hear this type of story almost every day from my patients. Too much motion and stress can lead to pain and joint damage. The difficulty is in determining just how much is "too much." A place to start in determining what is too much for you is related to the degree of lower-extremity arthritis or pathology that you have, as well as how you are coping with it. One person with knee pain from mild arthritis may be able to tolerate longer exercise sessions with a higher intensity than another. Someone who has more severe arthritis might not be able to tolerate more than ten minutes of low-intensity non-weight-bearing exercise.

You may need to see your orthopedic surgeon to determine how much arthritis you have. That information can help guide your selection of exercise type, duration, and intensity. If you do not consult with your orthopedist, then I recommend that you be conservative and err on the side of caution when it comes to developing your exercise program. In many cases, your doctor will confirm what you probably already suspect; in general, most people who have severe arthritis know it, although some may not want to admit it. Others may not fully comprehend the severity of their arthritis. I strongly recommend that you see your doctor. It's worth the time and money spent, especially if you are going to be serious about avoiding further injury and possible surgery. If you don't truly understand your degree of joint arthritis, the exercise program you chose could be riddled with problems. Knowing where you are starting will allow you to avoid the mistake of overdoing it and causing your joints to swell further.

Cross-training, not CrossFit, is a technique I like to recommend, because it can vary the load that exercise can put on joints. Cross-training is a way to work out that has you engage in a variety of exercises instead of only one. Each exercise stresses the joints in a different way, preventing joint overload. For example, you might bike for five minutes, speed walk for ten minutes, and do elliptical training for five minutes. It is better if you can do the exercises consecutively, one after the other, but spread them out if you can't fit them all in at one time on a particular day. Alternatively, instead of doing several different exercises on the same day, you can do a different exercise on different days of the week. Monday could be biking, Wednesday an exercise video, Friday the elliptical, and Saturday the treadmill. Ultimately, your joints will tell you when you have found the correct workout recipe. If your joints hurt or swell, then you need to alter what you are doing—either by identifying and eliminating the activity that is causing your pain or by doing your exercises less vigorously, for a shorter time period, or less frequently. By starting slowly, you'll minimize the chances of getting fired up to exercise and then being forced to stop due to pain and inflammation.

RESISTANCE TRAINING

When it comes to muscles, everybody wants to look good. My motto is: tone is good, maintaining strength is essential, and bulk is unnecessary. Strong muscles help joints track better, protect the joints against injury, and work like shock absorbers, protecting joints from stress. Muscles also consume calories like crazy. Increased muscle mass raises your basal metabolism. That means that when you're sitting on the couch, doing absolutely nothing, you're burning more calories if you have more muscle mass.

If your joints hurt, how do you go about strengthening your muscles? That is the million-dollar question, because your nervous system works against strengthening the muscles that surround painful joints. This concept is referred to as modulation of muscle recruitment. Let's look into this further.

Muscles work only when nerves tell them to. Have you ever tried to lift a lot of weight? In order to do it, you have to concentrate and direct your muscles to make a maximum effort. Olympic weight lifters get psyched up, approach the bar, breathe deeply, and explode into moving the weight. Their nerve endings offer 100 percent stimulation of the muscles via the maximum secretion of a molecular neurotransmitter called acetylcholine. A small amount of acetylcholine triggers a small muscular contraction, and a large amount results in a large contraction. As a form of self-preservation, to keep the muscles from overwhelming the damaged joint, the joint sends messages to the spinal cord to modulate or decrease the amount of acetylcholine or nerve stimulation that is sent to the muscles. Unfortunately, muscles that are chronically understimulated atrophy, or shrink in size. Smaller, atrophied muscles are weaker muscles. They don't protect the joint as well. They don't guide the joint effectively, nor do they burn calories or help control sugar levels. You do not want your muscles to atrophy.

People with arthritic joints have shrinking muscles that don't want to be stimulated. However, because you want to counter the atrophy, it is possible to stimulate a muscle that really doesn't want to be stimulated by controlling inflammatory signals. A well-devised and structured program with smart exercise, joint-healthy supplements, and an anti-inflammatory diet can be the answer. Exercising smart means choosing the muscles you need to strengthen, as well as using techniques that will build muscles without overloading your joints.

TYPES OF RESISTANCE TRAINING

When I was younger, I never heard of resistance training. Back then we called it *weight lifting*. Now I know that weight lifting is actually a type of resistance training using free weights or specially designed equipment. *Stretch band training,* sometimes called *resistance band training,* is another type of resistance training. A stretch band is used for resistance, instead of a barbell or specialized equipment. *Isometric* exercises are yet another type of resistance training, where the joint and muscles being trained are held in place and work statically. Put your hands in front of you like you are praying and push them together for five to ten seconds. That's isometric.

The diagrams below show examples of weight lifting, stretch band training, and isometric exercise.

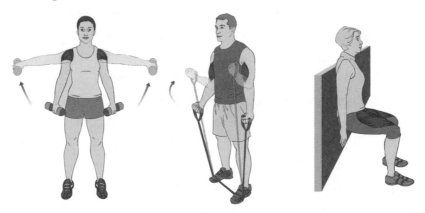

Knowing the various types of resistance training is important, because different severities of joint pain require different training techniques. Let's use the thigh muscle as an example. The thigh helps move the knee joint. With a minimally arthritic knee joint, the weight-lifting technique pictured below, called a leg extension, is an excellent way to develop thigh strength.

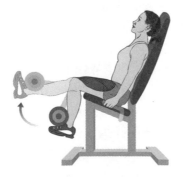

If the knee joint is more substantially arthritic or damaged, then the location of the structural problems needs to be taken into account. If grinding or pain occurs from 30 degrees to full extension, then this range of motion should be avoided. In this situation using stretch bands would be easier than using weights. The band would be adjusted to provide tension from about 110 degrees to just short of 30 degrees. The diagram below is an example of this technique.

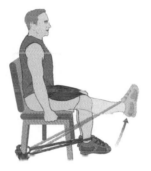

If the knee joint is damaged throughout, a mild isometric exercise, like a wall sit, can help strengthen the thigh without irritating the joint. A diagram of the wall sit is seen below. Having your knees bent at 90 degrees can be strenuous, so if you need to, stand more upright, with less bend in your knees. Remember to do only what you can tolerate. This isn't a competition. Typically you would per-form this exercise multiple times, holding for five to ten seconds longer as conditioning improves.

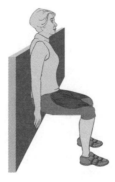

As you can see, if you wanted to use resistance training to strengthen your thighs, there are three options to choose from based on the severity of your knee arthritis. It is imperative that you determine the degree of arthritis affecting your joint and then apply the appropriate techniques for strengthening it. You can adjust which type of resistance training you use depending on your needs.

If you have severe knee arthritis, it might be necessary to use specially adapted isometric exercises for thigh and hamstring strengthening, but regular weight training might be perfectly fine for strengthening your shoulders, arms, and back. If you have severe arthritis, in general, you might consider weight training in warm water using waterproof weights that fasten with Velcro. The possibilities for how you can use resistance training are too numerous to detail individually. If you learn the principles of these methods of training and know your affected joints, then applying the correct techniques for you will be as easy as picking and choosing. You might use weights to strengthen joints with milder arthritis, resistance bands for more significant problems, and isometrics for the most severe problems. Remember that working in a limited range of motion is perfectly fine. Avoid the point at which grinding in the joint occurs, because that's where the arthritis is. Never forget the incredible magic of warm water as a place to get exercise (swimming), work your muscles (waterproof weights), and facilitate recovery (a warm bath or a whirlpool).

The exercises that follow are organized by body part and serve as examples of standard weight training, resistance band training, and isometric training. Suggestions for training frequency and repetitions (reps) will follow the diagrams. Assess the degree of arthritis for each body part, and pick the exercise that is appropriate (the exercises that follow are part of the eight-week program outlined in Part Two). If you have never done these exercises, you will need guidance to execute them properly. Find a trainer who can take you through the basics. There are a lot of video demonstrations on the internet, but be sure to train with a professional at least once to ensure proper form. Proceed with care and take this book with you. Strength will go hand in hand with joint relief and improved confidence. Have some fun. You can do it!

Biceps

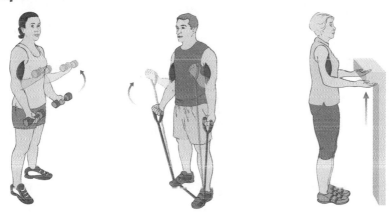

Triceps

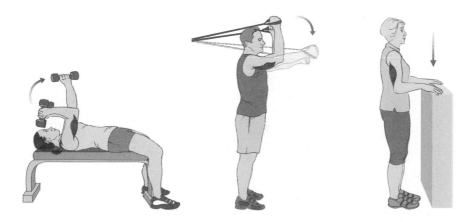

Shoulders

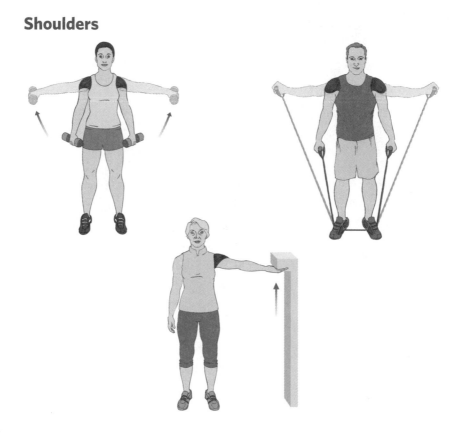

Chest

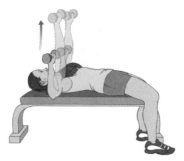

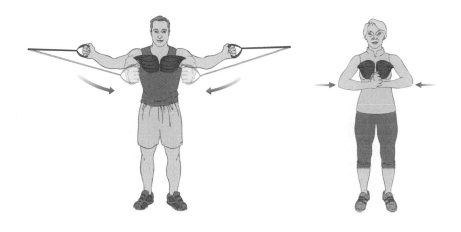

Upper Back

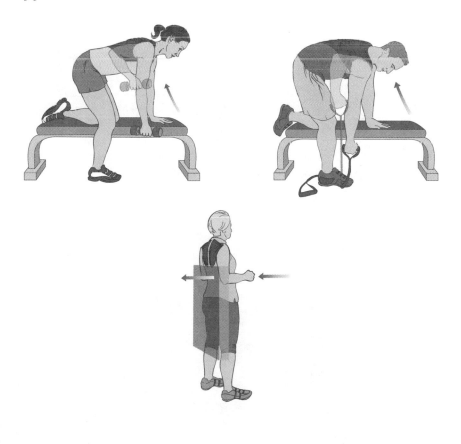

Lower Back

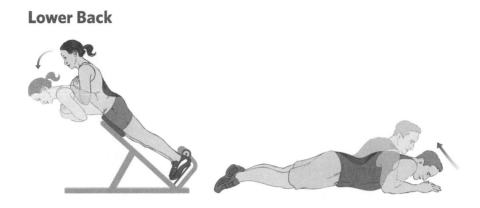

Thighs

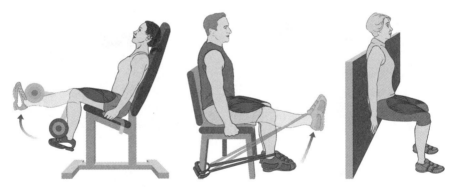

Hamstrings

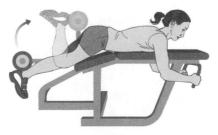

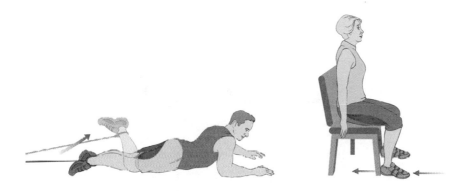

Calves

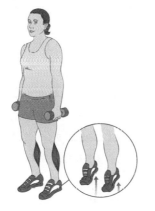

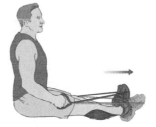

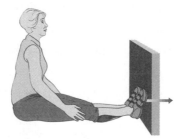

Abdominal

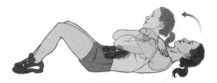

Spend about twenty minutes two times per week doing resistance training. Remember, when it comes to muscles, tone is good, strength is better, bulk is unnecessary. While I can't customize a program for each reader's joint pain, you can customize your program based on your needs. Some people will have only one joint that hurts, and others will have several. Limit your workout to two sets. You'll do one warm-up (lighter weight/resistance) and one live set (moderate weight/resistance). As you get better conditioned, you can warm up and then do two live sets of six to eight repetitions. When you are doing your resistance workout two times per week, you can do upper-body exercises one day and lower-body exercises the other day. I recommend that you do abdominal exercises each time you do your resistance training. Combine abs with your one day of upper-body training, as well as with your one day of lower-body training. Abdominal training, or core strengthening, also helps with back health, the area of the body that is most frequently injured. This workout schedule is not to train Olympians; it is to help strengthen your painful joints. While you strengthen your muscles, a host of very helpful structural and metabolic changes will take place.

A word of caution: Working out too much will counteract all the positive effects that you are attempting to achieve. Trust me, if you do too much, your joints will swell and you will feel it. If you are younger, are more vigorous, and have minimum pain, use your discretion and do more. Let your joints lead you.

CHOOSING YOUR WEIGHTS/RESISTANCE

It isn't necessary to do more intense training than what I suggest below unless you are training for a more athletic purpose. Light to moderate resistance is enough for joint health. Start out very light for safety reasons. Remember that different types of exercises will require different weight, e.g., five pounds for a curl and maybe fifty to one hundred pounds for a bench press.

- Lighter weight/resistance: You can easily do the recommended six to eight reps with no problem.
- Moderate weight/resistance: You need to work a bit to get through the reps, but not so much that you are struggling or can't complete the reps.

Resistance bands are typically color coded to designate the amount of force needed to move them. Start with the least amount of resistance and work your way up. The warm-up set is done with lighter weight/resistance and the second set is done with moderate weight/resistance.

DAY ONE		
Upper Body	Warm-Up Set (lighter weight/resistance)	Live Set (moderate weight/resistance)
Biceps	6–8 reps	6–8 reps
Triceps	6–8 reps	6–8 reps
Shoulders	6–8 reps	6–8 reps
Chest	6–8 reps	6–8 reps
Back	6–8 reps	6–8 reps
Abdomen	20 reps	20 reps

DAY TWO		
Lower Body	Warm-Up Set (lighter weight/resistance)	Live Set (moderate weight/resistance)
Thighs	6–8 reps	6–8 reps
Hamstrings	6–8 reps	6–8 reps
Calves	6–8 reps	6–8 reps
Abdomen	20 reps	20 reps

FLEXIBILITY TRAINING

Loss of range of motion leads to pain, which leads to immobility, which leads to more loss of range of motion. This is a predictable and debilitating path for those suffering with joint pain. As the joint becomes stiffer, increased forces are required to move an already injured and inadequate joint cartilage surface. The joint cartilage cannot absorb more stress and becomes overwhelmed and breaks down further (Smith 2000, 2004). Not only does function get worse as range of motion decreases, but also joint pain escalates, as the joint cartilage is subjected to increased stresses.

Flexibility allows for ease of movement and body control, and keeps the joints functioning well. Maintaining flexibility is essential for joint health. Flexibility protects the joint against heightened stresses, so the joint feels better. Flexibility fosters fluid joint function, making life easier. Time is of the essence. If you allow joint range of motion to diminish over an extended period of time and the ligaments become inflexible, you will experience more pain and potentially more damage to your joints.

Let's talk about the fundamentals of flexibility. The first thing to know is that the soft tissues (ligaments) surrounding your joints benefit from heat. If you take plastic outside into the freezing cold and bend it, it will snap. If you heat plastic over a gentle flame, it becomes supple and flexible. Relax. I'm not suggesting that you heat yourself up over a gentle flame, but I am suggesting that you need to warm up before stretching.

Two minutes on an exercise bike or a warm shower or bath are some gentle ways to warm up before stretching. Warm-water exercises are becoming popular in many parts of the country. With this technique, those with joint pain warm up and stretch in a 95°F to 100°F pool, taking advantage of the heat and the buoyancy of the water. Another example of an exercise that takes advantage of heat is Bikram yoga. This particular style of yoga is performed in 105°F heat and 40 percent humidity. Bikram yoga is an amazing workout, because you are stretching and strengthening at the same time. It can also be adapted to your joint needs and can be done vigorously or gently.

When you stretch, pay attention to pain and don't overstretch. The best approach is to perform stretches gently but firmly, with constant pressure, holding the stretch for a five- to ten-second count. No bouncing! That's how you hurt your joints. You need only to do five repetitions of each exercise, each with a five- to ten-second count, and you're all set. If you are stretching in order to maintain range of motion, a couple of times per week is plenty. If you have become stiff, you may need daily stretching sessions to regain your flexibility. If you have lost a lot of range of motion in a particular joint, you will most likely need help from an orthopedist and physical therapist to address your specific needs. However, because anyone can benefit from improved flexibility, I'll introduce you to some simple stretches that you can do to keep the primary joints of your body supple and fluid.

Neck

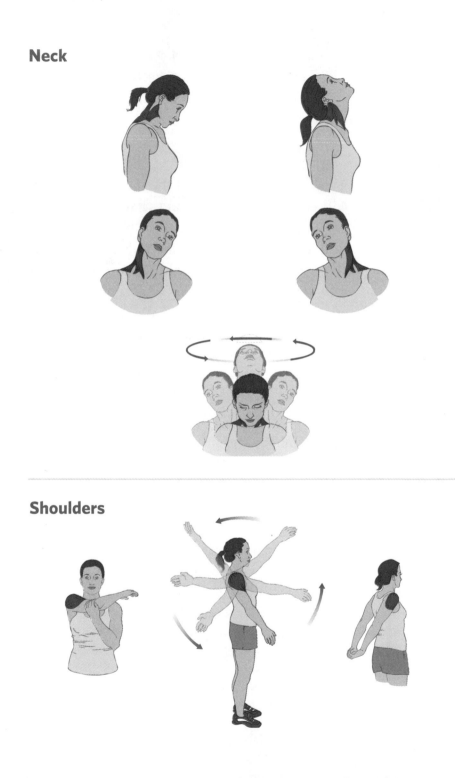

Shoulders

Elbows

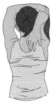
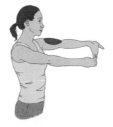

Wrists/Fingers

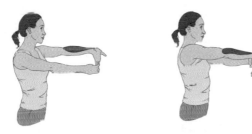

Back

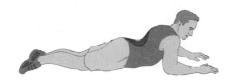

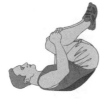
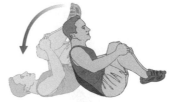

Thighs

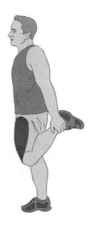

Hamstrings

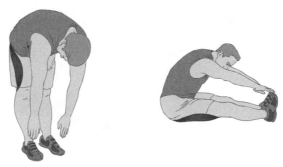

Groin

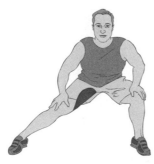
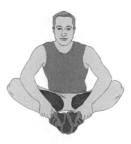

Calves and Achilles Tendons

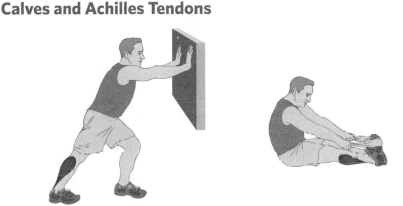

Ankles

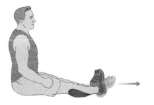

THE BEST-LAID PLANS

Everybody on our Yale football team liked one of our reserve kickers, Woody, but even more so, everybody respected him, because he was a hard worker. Each day he would show up for practice and kick field goals and extra points. He wasn't the starter, but that didn't stop him from preparing as if he were. We'd be on one side of the field, pounding one another, and Woody would be by himself, practicing literally thousands of kicks—kick after kick. He was like a machine.

The problem for Woody was that Tony, the guy playing in front of him, was really good. He was an accurate and powerful kicker with amazing range. Woody was never going to beat him out, but content in his role as a backup, Woody was ready to help the team if Tony ever got hurt.

As fate would have it, Tony never got hurt, but Woody got his chance to kick an extra point in one game. I remember the coach sending him in, and each one of us was excited that Woody was getting his opportunity. I can picture it like it was yesterday. The snap went down perfectly, the hold upright and steady, with laces forward, and the ball was ready for Woody to boot it through the uprights. He swung his leg smoothly, hit the football solidly, but unfortunately, he pulled the kick to the left. The referees signaled, "No good!" After thousands of practice kicks—*no good*. My heart dropped as Woody's head did the same.

He trotted off the field, clearly disappointed in the miss. None of us were disappointed in Woody, but we were all disappointed for him. As he scurried past Coach Cozza, lore has it that he said to Coach, "Guess I didn't practice enough." Can you imagine the fortitude to say after thousands of kicks, day after day, year after year, "Guess I didn't practice enough"? No excuses, curses, blame, or words of dejection. Simply, "Guess I didn't practice enough."

I'm telling you this story because life can be cruel. No matter how much you prepare, things don't always go the way you'd like them to. Look at Woody. But I love Woody's attitude, that way of thinking, *Things may not go right, but I am going to prepare and be as ready as humanly possible. I like my chances if I prepare for success.*

It's the same thing with joint health. Some people get dealt some terrible cards. They have bad genetics or simply bad luck. But that doesn't mean that you can't try your best to help yourself and let the chips fall as they may. Written on my high school locker-room wall was, "Luck is when opportunity meets preparation." I believe that following the *Healthy Joints for Life* program will swing luck in your direction.

Below, I've laid out the basic program so that you will be familiar with what I am going to ask you to do. The eight-week program will walk you through how to add exercise to your life.

THE *HEALTHY JOINTS FOR LIFE* EXERCISE PROGRAM	
Flexibility training	2x/week 10 minutes/session
Aerobic training	3x/week 20 minutes/session 5 minutes warm-up and stretch
Resistance training	2x/week 20–30 minutes/session

EXAMPLE SCHEDULE	
Monday	10 minutes warm-up and flexibility training 20 minutes aerobic training 30 minutes total
Tuesday	Rest
Wednesday	5 minutes warm-up 20 minutes aerobic training 30 minutes resistance training 55 minutes total
Thursday	Rest
Friday	Rest
Saturday	10 minutes warm-up and flexibility training 20 minutes aerobic training 30 minutes resistance training 60 minutes total

continued

EXAMPLE SCHEDULE	
Sunday	Rest
TOTAL TIME WORKING OUT	2 hours 25 minutes
TOTAL HOURS/WEEK	168 hours
TOTAL TIME TO REST	165 hours 35 minutes

In a single week I'm asking you to do 2 hours and 25 minutes of gentle working out and 165 hours and 35 minutes of rest. Does that put things into perspective?

WHERE DO WE GO FROM HERE?

We have already discussed the scientific evidence of the effects of diet, supplements, and exercise on NFkB, inflammation, and longevity, and you've officially formulated a well-thought-out game plan for joint health. Now that the game plan is in place, we need to prepare for game day. You are ready to embark on the eight-week program that will teach you to eat well, exercise smart, and supplement your joints to good health. It's game time!

PART TWO

The *Healthy Joints for Life* Program:

Eight Weeks to Reduce Pain and Inflammation

CHAPTER 6

READY:
Before You Begin

IN THE SAME WAY THAT YOU WOULDN'T GO ON A TRIP WITHOUT packing the appropriate clothes, you can't set out on the eight-week program to joint health without some prep work. You need to plan and prepare so that you will be ready for the dietary, supplement, and exercise changes that you will be making in your life.

In 1982, as an eager but scared twenty-one-year-old native New Englander, I set out for Miami to try out for the Miami Dolphins. You could think of my tryout as a six-week preseason program, two weeks shorter than your eight-week program to joint health.

Summer in New England was my favorite time of the year. I could do without the sweaters, parkas, and boots of winter. I loved the heat and humidity, but until I arrived in Miami in mid-July I didn't realize what stifling heat and humidity were. Now, that was real heat and humidity. The second you stepped out of the clubhouse door, the incredibly bright sun blinded you as it reflected off the white cement sidewalk. You would sweat during the twenty-yard walk to the practice field. People told me it wouldn't be so bad, it was a dry heat, no problem, and there was always a cool breeze. Clearly, they never practiced twice a day for six consecutive weeks wearing sweltering football equipment and a helmet. The heat wasn't dry, and there wasn't a breeze, ever. It didn't help that Coach Don Shula was scrutinizing every move I made.

The Dolphins provided everything I needed for their six-week preseason program. They had the appropriate clothes and equipment for me to wear. They provided us with supplements—salt pills—so we didn't become dehydrated. (You recall my Yale halftime story with the same salt pills. Sports medicine had some debatable thinking in those days.) And they had a wonderful nutrition program for me: weigh in every Monday at 218 pounds or get fined. Oddly enough, at that point in my life, football and that six-week preseason program were the only things that I really wanted to do. I endured the program, made the team, and together we battled all the way to the Super Bowl.

Your program is going to be much easier, because I won't be scrutinizing you or fining you. And I know this program is the only thing you're going to want to do, because you want your joints to feel better. You are going to win this battle.

Over the next eight weeks you are going to use diet, supplements, and exercise to reduce inflammation and control your joint pain. It will be a gradual program, which will begin with the slow introduction of correct food choices and eating habits. You will add supplements slowly over the same time frame. You will also gradually introduce and increase your exercise over the course of eight weeks. By the end of the eight weeks you will have a comprehensive program in place, and you should start to see significant results. By the end of six months the results should be life changing.

MY PATIENT VINNY

My late dad's name was Vinny, my older brother's name is Vinny, and his son's name... well, you guessed it... is Vinny, as well. I do not have a cousin named Vinny, in case you or Joe Pesci was wondering, but I do have a favorite patient named Vinny. He is sixty-seven-years-old, with an assortment of medical problems that prevent him from considering knee replacement surgery. His knees are bad; his cartilage is worn down, so that he has bone-on-bone pain. He can't take medications like Motrin, Naprosyn, or Celebrex because of an ulcer. I've used every trick in the trade to give him relief, from braces (which he hates) to shoe inserts to injections. He's grateful for everything I try. He uses a cane, but despite his pain, he doesn't like to complain.

I asked him to try my joint-healthy lifestyle program, and he smirked. I've seen that doubting smirk before. He wasn't ready, but over several months, as the pain escalated, my persistence and his near sense of futility made him agree to give it a try. At his one-month appointment he shrugged his shoulders when I inquired about his progress. I thought that he agreed to continue out of respect for me, but later, I found out it was because of desperation more than respect. He had no better options. By his three-month appointment he still limped but no longer used the cane. He came to that appointment with a homemade bottle of wine, my reward for his significant improvement.

PREPARING YOURSELF FOR SUCCESS

If you are anything like me, you have a few years of bad habits to break, habits that are directly causing you joint pain. Maybe you avoid exercise and can never say no to a piece of chocolate cake. Maybe you indulge in salty snacks, washed down with soda. Maybe you microwave frozen meals most days and don't have a fruit or vegetable as part of any meal. Don't beat yourself up about what has led you to the point of needing to correct your joint pain. What's done is done, and I'm going to give you the knowledge you need to move forward. You may have a few slips before you get into the swing of the program, and that's okay. You're only human. The trick is to keep your eye on your goals and always strive to achieve your best.

Your dietary goals over the next eight weeks are:

- Minimize carbs
- Maximize fiber
- Eat colorful fruits and vegetables
- Eat the right protein
- Avoid trans fats and unhealthy saturated fats
- Maximize omega-3 fats and minimize omega-6s
- Eat fats in combination with proteins and carbs to slow carb absorption
- Eat frequently to prevent uncontrolled hunger
- Eat sensible portions
- Find healthy alternatives for dietary pitfalls

PUTTING YOUR KITCHEN ON A DIET (OR EXORCISING THE JOINT DEVILS)

Before we discuss exercising for joint health, we need to discuss exorcising the joint devils from your kitchen and pantry. Your absolute first step to appropriate nutrition must be to get your kitchen and fridge into joint-healthy shape. Having the temptations of *joint devils* lurking on every shelf of the refrigerator and in every corner of the pantry will only lead to failure. Joint devils are those foods that contribute to joint pain and trigger NFkB and all its inflammatory partners in crime. They are also foods that contribute to cardiovascular disease and diabetes, among other diseases, so it's a good thing to get them out of your house. It is going to take some discipline, but you have to get rid of the high carbohydrate–, high salt–, unhealthy trans fat–, and saturated fat–laden foods that fill your kitchen and are murder on your joints.

At first, you may encounter resistance from a family member— your wife, husband, daughter, son, or mother-in-law. Pasta, chips, beer, and sweets are quite addicting, and they might not be willing to give them up . . . yet. Use your powers of persuasion to get friends and family on board to become partners in your quest for better health. Remind them that if you are able to move more freely, then you will be a better husband, wife, or friend, and you will be happier and will be able to spend time with them in the activities you all enjoy. And while they may not be suffering from joint pain, the foods you will be filling your kitchen with have many other benefits, such as reducing heart disease and cancer risks and more. Anyone can benefit from healthier eating. Remember, if you keep some chips in the house "for your guests" or "for the kids," you will undoubtedly eat them at some point. Get rid of them. The program will provide replacements that your guests will enjoy equally. Let me give you a great example.

It was an early fall Sunday afternoon, and my wife had just left to visit her mom and dad. My daughter and son were both out with their friends. I was home by myself and excited at the prospect of an afternoon of NFL football. Maybe that's not your cup of tea, but for me, it's better than being on the French Riviera. Well, not quite that good, but darn close.

I headed to the family room, grabbed the remote, and turned on the TV, complete with surround sound. The team uniform colors exploded across the screen amid the cheers of the crowd. Once the TV was set up, I went to the pantry in search of a drink and a snack. Perhaps I would have some nachos and a beer, or wings and a Coke, or chips or Fritos and dip. I was heading toward snacking myself into an unnecessary state of inflammation and joint pain.

While my head danced with visions of crispy trans fats, lucky for me, the pantry had been cleansed of temptation. There were no inflammation-provoking, fat-forming snacks to be found. Instead, there were plenty of joint-healthy alternatives. I chose sliced cucumbers with hummus and four ounces of mangosteen juice mixed into a tall glass of ice-cold seltzer. I loaded up a low-carb pita with sliced chicken and pesto. It was all delicious and satisfying. I was in heaven and my joints were, too.

FROM THE PANTRY

Remove (or donate) canned soups, cereals, high-carb pastas and breads, jars of tomato sauce, cake mixes, frosting, chips, pretzels, popcorn, crackers, cookies, granola, granola bars, tacos, dried fruit, canola oil and other vegetable oils, barbecue sauce, and candy.

FROM THE FRIDGE AND FREEZER

Remove salad dressings, fruit juices, barbecue sauce, ketchup, maple syrup, jelly, jam, ice cream toppings, frozen pizza, ready-to-eat meals, processed lunch meats, high-sugar yogurt, and all the left over Chinese food and other fat-laden foods. (There are some healthier versions of dressings and sauces, but you need to look carefully at the label.)

LOOK FOR THE (JOINT) DEVIL IN THE DETAILS ON THE LABEL

Ingredients to watch for on any food package label include high fructose corn syrup (HFCS), corn syrup, and corn syrup solids. Here's something you might find interesting: Corn syrup is liquid, obviously, and the sugar in it is glucose (aka dextrose), so corn syrup is still sugar. Corn syrup solids are corn syrup without the water, so its like concentrated corn syrup in powder form. HFCS is corn syrup enzymatically changed to have fructose instead of the glucose, so it is sweeter.

Other sugars/sweeteners include dextrose (glucose), table sugar (sucrose), fructose, honey, and molasses. Most people don't know that molasses is made by boiling the sweet juice extracted from sugarcane plants or sugar beets. The juice undergoes several rounds of boiling, and during the process sugar is extracted from it. The first boiling produces light molasses, which is sweeter than the molasses that results from the second or third boiling. A second boiling yields dark molasses, and a third boiling blackstrap molasses, which is the kind used in foods like baked beans. The darker the molasses, the less sugar it contains. Sulfur dioxide is sometimes added as a preservative if the plants are less mature and green when harvested. Mature plants need not be treated, since they do not spoil.

Check out the label on every item on the pantry shelves and toss those that contain finely ground flour, regardless of whether it is wheat, bleached, unbleached, enriched, or rice. You should stay away from trans fats, partially hydrogenated oils, vegetable oils (soybean is a commonly used bad oil, with omega-6s, remember?), and glycerin (this is the backbone of triglycerides, which are especially unhealthy for the cardiovascular system).

LEARNING HOW TO SHOP

The first step in finding healthy (and tasty) alternatives for the foods that will invariably lead to joint pain is to change the way you shop.

You will learn to stay away from packaged foods and highly processed foods and to gravitate to joint-healthy alternatives. You will be
replacing inflammation-supporting, NFkB-friendly foods with those
that combat inflammation and NFkB on a cellular level: vegetables
full of vitamins and phytonutrients (zucchini, red peppers, mushrooms, and more), seasonings that liven up your meals and please
your palate (including ginger, garlic, and cinnamon), dairy products
that contain healthy fats to slow carbohydrate absorption (cottage
cheese, yogurt, and mozzarella cheese), fruits that are full of nutrients and fiber (such as apples, avocados, and pomegranates), beans
that are packed with protein and fiber (like chickpeas, kidney beans,
and lentils), breads and pastas that are tasty and low carb (such as
pumpernickel bread, whole wheat bread and pasta, and egg fettuccine), and proteins that are the mainstay of any anti-inflammatory
diet (including salmon, lobster, and grass-fed beef). Learning how
to be joint healthy makes grocery shopping much more enjoyable.
There is an incredible "pride in ownership" feeling when your grocery
cart is full of colorful and healthy foods. You know you are helping
yourself and your family to eat better and feel better. Be imagina-
tive. Be willing to try something new and your joints will thank you.

VEGETABLES
Vegetables are teeming with incredible vitamins and phytonutrients.
The brighter the colors of the vegetables, the better they are for you.
While you're shopping, imagine expanding your palate with a kale
salad mixed with slivers of red pepper, cucumber, and onion. Think
about a healthy stir-fry of broccoli and mushrooms in coconut oil
for a delicious side dish. Sprouts in salads and on sandwiches add
a delightful crunch and are especially helpful for women with hot
flashes and PMS. Try an omelet with scallions and sprouts. Don't
be afraid to experiment! Shopping, especially in anticipation of the
delicious foods you will be eating, should be fun!

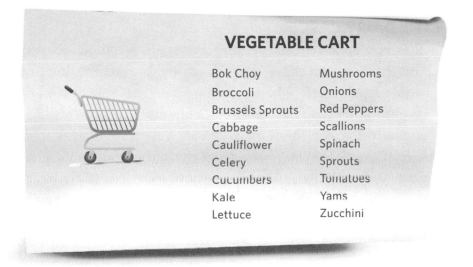

VEGETABLE CART

Bok Choy	Mushrooms
Broccoli	Onions
Brussels Sprouts	Red Peppers
Cabbage	Scallions
Cauliflower	Spinach
Celery	Sprouts
Cucumbers	Tomatoes
Kale	Yams
Lettuce	Zucchini

THE SPICE OF LIFE

Seasonings are the spice of life. They liven up every dish, and the seasonings listed below are joint healthy, so use them liberally. You can't eat enough turmeric and ginger. Baked broccoli with olive oil and garlic is incredible. I could eat it every night. Oregano has an incredible ORAC value to fight free radicals. Check out how my wife prepares roasted chicken with rosemary and thyme (see pages 80–81), a dish that packs a protein punch and is tasty, too!

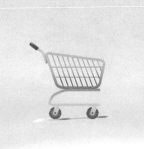

SEASONING CART

Basil	Ginger
Black Pepper	Green Tea
Chili	Oregano
Cilantro	Parsley
Cinnamon	Rosemary
Cumin	Turmeric
Dark Cocoa	Thyme
Garlic	

IN THE DAIRY CASE

A dollop of whipped cream over berries, stevia-sweetened yogurt, and cottage or ricotta cheese can be healthy desserts for those of you with a sweet tooth. Add dark cocoa powder to a small bowl of ricotta cheese to make chocolate ricotta pudding. You won't be disappointed. You may be more accustomed to skim milk rather than whole milk, or vice versa. I like having the extra fat of whole milk because it slows down carb absorption. Whole milk or skim milk is acceptable in small quantities—the quantity is important. Milk sugar is lactose, which is a glucose molecule connected to a galactose molecule. Break it down and you have glucose, which will give you an insulin spike. Keep the consumption of milk below one cup per day, which is twelve grams of carbs. Butter doesn't have the best fat profile, but if you use it in smaller quantities, it can be acceptable. Less than one tablespoon is one hundred calories and seven grams of saturated fat. Ironically, low-fat yogurts usually have a higher sugar content, so regular yogurt is probably a better choice, although regular yogurt with fruit on the bottom can pack a lot of sugar. Make checking labels a habit.

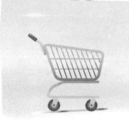

DAIRY PRODUCT CART

Cottage Cheese	Plain Yogurt
Low-Sugar Ice Cream (no sugar added)	Ricotta Cheese
	Whipped Cream
Mozzarella Cheese	Whole Milk

FRESH FRUIT

I have a tree fruit allergy, so I can't eat raw tree fruits, but I can eat tree fruits if they are cooked. Apparently, the cooking process changes the shape of the molecules in the fruit that I'm allergic to, so my body no longer recognizes them as foreign. (You knew I would explain that, didn't you?) That's why I love baked apples with cinnamon. I also love berries, especially blackberries. And grapefruit is spectacular sprinkled with Truvia, a brand of stevia. Avocado is a fruit, although I usually eat it like a vegetable on sandwiches or in guacamole with onions. Pomegranates can brighten up any plate and are especially joint healthy. Remember, fruit is tasty because it is full of natural sugar, and although the sugar is natural, it is still sugar, so portions have to be watched closely. Note that I recommend red grapes over white, because it is the skin of the red grape that has all the good nutrients.

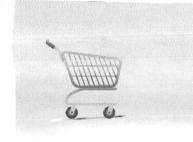

FRUIT CART

Apples	Grapefruit
Avocado	Pomegranates
Blackberries	Raspberries
Blueberries	Red Grapes
Cherries	Strawberries

A BOUNTY OF BEANS

Don't underestimate the protein and fiber you get from beans. Ground cooked chickpeas are used to make hummus, which is a delicious dip, and ground dried chickpeas constitute a low-carb flour. Lentil soup is filling and full of fiber. I have a weakness for chili, so I can't recommend kidney beans more heartily.

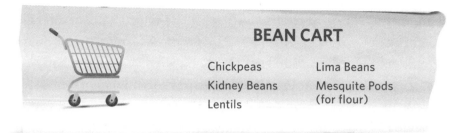

BEAN CART

Chickpeas	Lima Beans
Kidney Beans	Mesquite Pods
Lentils	(for flour)

GOOD GRAINS AND SEEDS

If you don't give barley a chance, you are making a big mistake. It is fantastic in soups and can be ground into a low-carb flour and then used to make healthy scones and muffins. Barley has beta-glucan, a variety of soluble fiber that is great for slowing carb absorption. Buckwheat is high in protein and soluble fiber. Buckwheat is a pseudocereal, not a grain, but for the purposes of this book, I include it in the commentary on grain. It reduces cholesterol and blood pressure. Kasha, made from buckwheat kernels, is a popular Eastern European cereal. Buckwheat is a versatile "grain" and can be combined with milk and cinnamon for a delicious dessert porridge or with onions, scallions, and olive oil as an entrée side dish. Don't forget that grains are carbs and you don't want to eat lots of carbs. Barley added to soup is great, because only a small quantity is needed and it is very tasty!

Brown rice is better than white, because it has more fiber and a lower GI, but you can't forget that rice is a carb and that it's best to minimize its consumption. Steel-cut oats have a much lower GI than instant oatmeal, which you should avoid. Try cooking the oats a bit less than suggested. This helps lower the GI, as well. Like buckwheat, quinoa is technically not a grain, but it's close enough, so it is included in the grain section. Quinoa is a compromise to vegetarians, which I vacillate on. It does provide nutrients and some protein, but it also is a predominant carb source, so eat it in smaller quantities. Whole wheat kernels can give a nice texture to foods—½ cup cooked whole wheat kernels provide ten grams of carbs and only two grams of protein. The GI of whole-kernel wheat is much lower (as low as 30) than that of cracked wheat (48) or finely ground wheat (85).

Flaxseed is my favorite seed because the body can turn it into large quantities of omega-3s, it's full of fiber, and it has almost as much protein as carbohydrate. I treat it like oatmeal, putting it in boiling water to cook like a cereal and then topping it with cinnamon. Delicious.

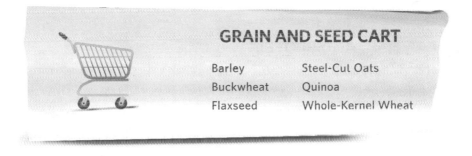

GRAIN AND SEED CART

Barley	Steel-Cut Oats
Buckwheat	Quinoa
Flaxseed	Whole-Kernel Wheat

BREADS AND PASTAS

Breads and pastas can be joint killers, especially those made with finely ground flour. It is when flour is finely ground that it is a problem, so look for whole grain for joint health. I used to be a big sandwich eater, but once I realized what all that bread was doing to my joints, that changed. Now I love low-carb, whole-grain pita pockets, which have only five grams of carbs! Fill a pocket with some diced chicken, mozzarella, sprouts, olive oil, and turmeric and you have a scrumptious sandwich that will soothe your joints. Low-carb pastas and egg pastas are great with garlic-infused tomato sauce. Just remember to eat moderate portions because of the glycemic load. A couple of hints about pasta: The GI of pasta is lower if you cook it al dente. Eating pasta cold also lowers the GI. Cold al dente pasta salad is, therefore, the best!

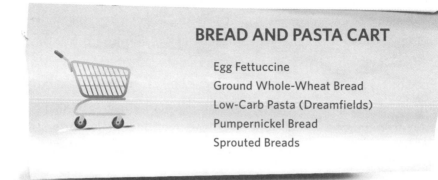

BREAD AND PASTA CART

Egg Fettuccine

Ground Whole-Wheat Bread

Low-Carb Pasta (Dreamfields)

Pumpernickel Bread

Sprouted Breads

MEAT, FISH, AND PROTEIN

Protein is a mainstay of any anti-inflammatory diet. Lower saturated fat protein sources are preferred, unless the saturated fats tend toward stearic fatty acid, found in grass-fed beef, which is joint healthy.

Pay a little more for your protein sources and they'll taste better and be joint healthier. A small piece of grass-fed beef with a grilled lobster tail, and you are eating as well as a king! Don't forget to consider protein powders: whey for faster absorption and casein for slower absorption. Try my favorite "on the go" smoothie by combining in a blender a fiber powder like Metamucil, the protein powder of your choice, ice cubes, a teaspoon of yogurt, a few berries and blending until smooth.

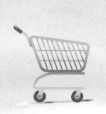

PROTEIN CART

Buffalo	Mackerel
Chicken	Pork Chops
Eggs	Protein Powder
Fish (in general)	(whey and casein)
Grass-Fed Beef	Turkey
Lobster	Wild Alaskan Sockeye Salmon

A SPOONFUL OF _____

The ultimate objective should be to reduce your use of sweeteners as much as possible. When your sweet tooth gets the best of you, turn to stevia first. If that's not available, then use Splenda, a sucralose-based artificial sweetener. Although I'm not a big proponent of Splenda, it's better than Equal, which contains aspartame, a sweetener that has a checkered reputation since it breaks down into wood alcohol and formaldehyde, which are both known toxins. I do not like it from a metabolic standpoint. Honey (containing the sugars fructose and glucose predominantly) has a delicious flavor, and if you're going to indulge on occasion, it's better than other sugars, including table sugar, fructose, and agave, which breaks down into fructose. You may recall that fructose binds exceptionally well to collagen, which causes joint ligaments and cartilage to become stiff. (Various Australian honeys have been tested for GI and the following are all considered low GI (35-52): Yellow Box, Stringybark, Red Gum, Iron Bark, and Yapunyah.)[*] Honey GI is most related to fructose/glucose ratio. Higher fructose content leads to lower GI which is good for insulin response but bad for glycation of collagen and triglyceride production.

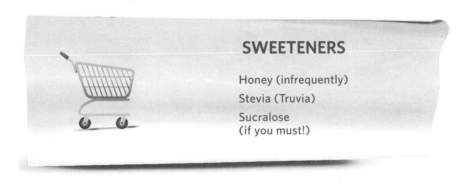

SWEETENERS

Honey (infrequently)

Stevia (Truvia)

Sucralose
(if you must!)

---

[*] "A Preliminary Assessment of the Glycemic Index of Honey: A Report for the Australian Rural Industries Research and Development Corporation" by Dr. Jayashree Arcot and Prof Jennie Brand-Miller

BEVERAGES

Remember to drink seventy-two ounces of water per day. You don't have to drink only pure water. Seltzer, green tea, hot chocolate with Truvia, various juices in small quantities, such as mangosteen juice, ice-based smoothies, and protein shakes are great sources of water. If you can't live without coffee, I recommend that you try to wean yourself off it and substitute tea instead. Green tea is best, but black tea is certainly better than coffee. Buy a mini-blender with detachable cups so you can blend your drink and take it with you. Invest in a seltzer machine for the variety and fun of it. Don't drink soda! Sodas, teeming with phosphoric acid, leach calcium from your bones.

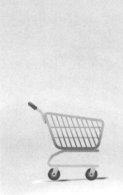

BEVERAGE CART
(including all supplies to make beverages)

Alcohol (light beer and red wine are on hold for the first eight weeks)

Berries (for smoothies)

Black Tea

Blender

Cocoa Powder (unsweetened dark for hot chocolate)

Green Tea

Mangosteen Juice

Seltzer Machine

Water

Waters, Flavored (occasionally)

Yogurt (unsweetened for smoothies)

INFLAMMATION-FREE DINING

Below you will find a brief overview of food and drink suggestions that will point you in the right direction when it comes to meal preparation. I hope these lists will jump-start your imagination. There are some foods here that you shouldn't miss, as well as some foods you might enjoy making and love eating. You may discover a new food or combination of foods that you hadn't been aware of but that will certainly be something good to add to your table.

Breakfast Ideas

Turkey bacon

Berry smoothie with yogurt

Fried egg sandwich on low-carb pita

Omelet with spinach, peppers, scallions, and mushrooms
    (use whole eggs and egg whites)

Scrambled eggs with mozzarella cheese

Flaxseed porridge with cinnamon and raw apple pieces

Grapefruit (½ cup) with Truvia (skip the juice)

Lox on a low-carb pita with scallions and capers

Oatmeal (steel-cut oats)

Toasted sprouted bread with a teaspoon of natural peanut
    butter and a cup of tea

Yogurt (unsweetened variety)

Lunch or Dinner Ideas

Pesto chicken with julienned summer squash

Panfried pork chops with peppers, onions, and cherry peppers

Grilled buffalo steaks

Grilled grass-fed beef

Turkey or chicken burgers with cheese and avocado

Sautéed grass-fed beef strips with scallions

Baked chicken with olive oil, rosemary, and thyme

Buffalo meatballs and tomato sauce with basil over low-
    carb pasta

Sautéed salmon with capers and diced tomatoes

Baked or sautéed flounder with wasabi-flavored light
olive oil mayonnaise

Vegetables

Grilled zucchini drizzled with olive oil
Sautéed peppers and scallions
Kale, broccoli rabe, or bok choy sautéed with garlic
Baked or steamed broccoli with olive oil and lemon
Mashed cauliflower
Stewed chickpeas with lentils and barley
Sautéed tomatoes and onions or scallions with olive oil
Sautéed mushrooms
Baked yams
Cole slaw with minimal carrots and light
olive oil mayonnaise
Baked and browned Brussels sprouts

Desserts

Ricotta with cocoa powder sweetened with Truvia
Fresh berries with whipped cream
Chocolate-dipped strawberries (sugar free)
Jell-O or pudding (sugar free)
Baked apples with cinnamon
Dark chocolate (sugar free)
Blackberry sorbet (sugar free)
Coconut macaroon cookies (sugar free)
Oatmeal chocolate chip cookies (sugar free)
Cheesecake with pecan crust
Peanut butter balls

Beverages

Green tea (hot or cold)

Ginger, pomegranate, pineapple, and cranberry refresher
(a flavoring in seltzer)

Mangosteen juice shot over ice

Lemonade slushie with Truvia

Fruit smoothie with yogurt

Chocolate or vanilla protein shake

Hot chocolate made with unsweetened dark chocolate
and Truvia

Seltzer (flavored or not)

Water

Red wine (on occasion, but not during the eight weeks
of the program)

Light beer (on occasion, but not during the eight weeks
of the program)

SELECTING SUPPLEMENTS

The supplement aisle can be overwhelming, so I will help clarify what the labels mean and what to look for to be sure you are not only getting the most potent bang for your buck but are also selecting the correct type of supplements and vitamins to combat joint pain and inflammation most effectively. What these supplements will do for you:

- Provide antioxidants
- Reduce free radicals
- Bolster bone, ligament, and cartilage health
- Reduce inflammation through a variety of pathways
- Facilitate weight loss

- Improve energy level
- Reduce joint pain

The supplements listed below will be added to your regimen over the course of the eight weeks. By taking a slow approach to adding supplements, you can determine what works best for you based on your tolerance of a particular supplement. I take all these supplements and tolerate them perfectly well, but you will need to take it as it goes. Not all supplements are created equal. It is best to purchase from a manufacturer that tests each batch of supplements with an independent company. This will be noted on the bottle. You may also see a label from, for example, ConsumerLab.com, NSF International, or the United States Pharmacopeial Convention, all of which have a dietary supplement certification program. Keep in mind that the least expensive supplement is not always the best choice.

WHAT DO THE LABELS MEAN?

When shopping for supplements and vitamins, it is important that you look at the labels before you buy. Not only do you want to ensure that you are purchasing the proper dosage, but you want to be certain that you are buying quality supplements and vitamins.

You should look for the active ingredient, the quantity of active ingredient in each tablet or capsule, and any validation stamp.

HEALTHY JOINTS FOR LIFE SUPPLEMENT STACK	
SUPPLEMENT	RECOMMENDED DAILY DOSAGE*
Lutein	10–40 mg 1x/day
Astaxanthin	2–4 mg 1x/day
Vitamin B_6	10–20 mg 1x/day
Vitamin B total mixed	Multi of B_1–B_{12} 1x/day
Vitamin C	500 mg 2x/day
Vitamin D_3	2000–5000 IU 1x/day
Vitamin E total mixed	100 IU 1x/day
Vitamin E gamma-tocotrienol	15 mg 1x/day
Calcium	250 mg 2x/day
Omega-3s	1000 mg 2x/day
PAC/Grape seed extract	200 mg 2x/day
Resveratrol	250 mg 1x/day
Curcumin (biocurcumax)	250–500 mg 2x/day
Boswellia	300 mg 2x/day
Pomegranate extract	250–500 mg 2x/day
Ginger	500–1000 mg 1x/day
Green tea	270 mg total EGCG in 2–3 separate doses
Glucosamine	1500 mg 1x/day
Chondroitin	1200 mg 1x/day
Licorice root (max 1-month cycle)	400 mg of glycyrrhizic acid 1x/day (maximum dose)
NAC	600 mg 1x/day
Silymarin	200 mg 2x/day

* Dosages of proprietary supplements with improved absorption can be lessened

A note on multivitamins: While it is perfectly okay to take a multivitamin, there is no multivitamin available that has all these supplements at the recommended dosages. The pill necessary to include everything would be too big to swallow! You can look carefully at the label and find various combination products, but there isn't a single capsule that contains all the recommended supplements. It will be necessary for you to take individual or combination supplements, rather than a single multivitamin/supplement, in order to get the dosages I recommend. Some of the supplements, such as the B vitamins, B_1 to B_{12}, and the E vitamins, tocopherols and tocotrienols, come in combination form. Another example is resveratrol, which comes in combination with curcumin in some preparations. Dosages also depend on patient weight as well as supplement bioavailability. A 110 pound person does not need the same dosage as a 250 pound person. Similarly BCM-95 curcumin with several-fold improved bioavailability need not be dosed as high as regular curcumin. Visit www.healthyjointsforlife.com for easy options and insight on the most appropriate supplements.

BEFORE YOU MOVE A MUSCLE

Once the kitchen is sorted and you've selected your supplements, it's time to focus on what you need to exercise effectively and efficiently. This is highly individualized. For some it will mean designating a place in your home where you will use exercise DVDs, for others it will mean buying new sneakers so you can walk comfortably, and for others it will mean signing up for a gym membership. Make sure you have the location, the equipment, and the commitment to do your exercise program.

Commitment can be the hardest part. If you feel pain in your joints when you exercise or even during the course of a normal day, you may be reluctant to exercise. You'll need to trust me on this one: once you get moving, your joints will feel better. You can let pain be your guide. I certainly don't expect you to push through tortuous pain. I would much prefer that you do as much as is comfortable, with the expectation of doing more in the future. Doing just a little is better than doing nothing. Establish a strategy to stick with exercising. For instance, set aside a few minutes in your day. Make an appointment with yourself to exercise, and physically write it in your calendar or enter it into your smartphone. Make a plan to work out with someone else for a specific day and time—their encouragement and effort to keep the date and to stick with the exercise plan could be all the support that's necessary!

What your exercise program will do for you:

- Gently stress joints to strengthen muscles and bones
- Improve lubrication in your joints
- Stretch to maintain flexibility and joint range of motion
- Improve conditioning or exercise tolerance, so exercise becomes easier

WHAT YOU ARE GOING TO NEED
TO EXERCISE: THE BARE MINIMUM

For the three most basic components of the joint-healthy exercise program, namely, walking, isometric exercising, and stretching, you will need only sturdy walking shoes and loose-fitting clothing.

You will need additional equipment as you increase your aerobic activity, strength training, and stretching. Most of the equipment mentioned in this chapter can be found in a gym or is available in a group class. A gym will have exercise machines that are geared toward strengthening and toning specific muscles and body parts. If you are so inclined, you can purchase exercise equipment to use in your own home. If you were going to invest in one piece of equipment, I would suggest something for aerobic conditioning and would tailor it to the joints involved and your severity of arthritis: a treadmill for mild arthritis, an elliptical machine or stationary bike for moderate arthritis, and a stationary bike for severe arthritis.

WHAT YOU ARE GOING TO NEED
TO EXERCISE: THE NEXT STEP UP

Weight training: exercise bands of various strengths (they are usually color coordinated to indicate the level of resistance), handheld weights of various weights, and, most likely, a gym membership.

Stretching: a yoga mat and the diagrams shown here for the stretching exercises. If you prefer, you could substitute a yoga DVD or a Pilates DVD for my stretches. If you haven't done either of these types of exercises before, start with a beginner program and work your way up to more advanced poses and movements. Keep in mind that yoga and Pilates movements are more advanced stretching activities than my basic stretches. If you are particularly stiff, my stretches are a good starting point.

Aerobic exercise: workout DVDs, sports equipment (for the sport of your choice, such as tennis or golf), a stationary bike, a road/trail bike, an elliptical machine, a treadmill, a jump rope, running shoes, and any sport-specific workout gear/clothing.

***

Now that your kitchen is in order, you have your supply of supplements, and you are prepared to work out, it's time to get started on your *Healthy Joints for Life* eight-week program.

CHAPTER 7

WEEK ONE:
Healthy Joints for Life

EAT

GETTING ON SCHEDULE

THIS FIRST WEEK ESTABLISHES THE HABIT OF EATING EVERY THREE to four hours. Not only will eating this way keep your appetite in check and prevent you from becoming uncontrollably hungry, but it will also continually replenish the essential nutrients necessary to maintain healthy joints and control inflammation. As a general guideline, I suggest eating breakfast at 8:00 a.m., a snack at 10:00 a.m., lunch at noon, a second snack at 3:00 p.m., and then dinner between 6:00 and 7:00 p.m., with a delayed dessert or snack at about 9:00 p.m. Naturally, those times can be slightly adjusted to your specific lifestyle. In later weeks we are going to introduce a pre-bedtime snack.

The first week focuses on establishing the schedule and getting you to eat more often than you are accustomed to. Oddly enough, eating more frequently will ultimately decrease the amount that you eat by controlling your hunger. With your pantry and fridge set up to be free of joint devils, the only things you'll be able to eat will be good foods. For the time being, we are not going to worry too much about portions, calories, and so on. I'd really like you to get used to eating these great foods on a schedule. We'll be refining the amounts you will eat in week seven.

If you work outside of your home, then at least three of the six meals or snacks you eat will probably be at work. Get yourself an inexpensive insulated lunch box and bring your healthy lunch and snacks with you to work so you can keep your drinks cool and food warm or cold. Remember, enjoying the food you eat will be important for your success. By bringing food from home, you will not be tempted to run out to the deli or food cart or to a fast-food restaurant to get what would undoubtedly be a less than joint-friendly meal. Your joints can't afford to dine out on standard fare yet. Remember, you are what you eat: Every bad fat that you eat ends up in your cell membranes and can then be converted into an inflammatory molecule. This leads to joint pain.

In the beginning of the eight-week program, you need to stock your cell membranes with all the right "stuff." No exceptions. If work necessitates that you eat out with clients, then eat smart! Stay away from fried foods, which will undoubtedly provide saturated fats and will probably supply trans fats. Choose the right protein source: grilled chicken instead of sliced grilled steak, turkey instead of salami. Choose your side dish wisely, for instance, a salad sprinkled with olive oil, instead of potato chips or fries. Brightly colored vegetables contain healthy nutrients and antioxidants that fight inflammation. Low-glycemic carbs are a must. Stay away from the cheeseburger (bad fat) on the kaiser roll (bad carbs). Eat salmon with broccoli instead of a BLT. And don't allow condiments and sauces to sabotage an otherwise great meal. Ketchup made with high fructose corn syrup could spoil the positive effects of a bison burger. Hollandaise sauce would ruin a perfectly fine poached egg on a thin slice of sprouted bread.

It is important to establish a pattern and a schedule of eating that will become second nature. I've found that most patients do fine in the morning but run into trouble in the afternoon and at nighttime (primarily due to hunger). The morning snack that I recommend is important to keep sugar/insulin levels steady so that hunger spikes don't occur near lunchtime. Similarly, the afternoon snack keeps hunger spikes at bay so you don't become ravenous around dinnertime. A packaged mozzarella stick or a low-carb protein bar can be worked into virtually any lifestyle and can be the perfect remedy to hunger spikes.

Don't get overly concerned about what you are eating as long as it's directly from your newly stocked pantry and fridge. Focus on getting used to eating frequently. Become comfortable with the idea of preparing ahead of time what you are going to eat while at work. Establish the hourly intervals between meals and snacks, which are necessary to alleviate uncontrolled hunger.

MEAL SCHEDULE	
8:00 a.m.–9:00 a.m.	Breakfast
Midmorning	Snack (if breakfast is eaten before 8:00 a.m. or if hunger mounts)
12:00 p.m.–1:00 p.m.	Lunch
3:00 p.m.	Snack
6:00 p.m.–7:00 p.m.	Dinner
8:00 p.m.–9:00 p.m.	Snack or Low-carb dessert

SUPPLEMENT

INTRODUCING LEVEL I SUPPLEMENTS

Chapter 4 and Appendix I present the scientific basis for taking supplements for joint-pain relief. I take each and every supplement mentioned below daily, but that may not work with your finances or for your personal situation. To accommodate individual needs, I've arranged the supplements according to four levels. Naturally, you should purchase supplements as your budget allows. No doctor or supplement expert can predict which individual supplement or group of supplements will be most effective for a specific person. If each supplement is scientifically backed, then it makes sense to try as many as possible and see which ones work.

Level I supplements are not "better" than those of any other level. However, I do believe this level represents a gold standard that everyone should adopt. I've diversified the levels to include vitamins and supplements that fight inflammation in different ways. It is my hope that you will follow my lead and take all the supplements I recommend; however, I completely understand if that is not possible. The program eases you into each supplement level. This will allow you to determine how well each level is tolerated. If you take all four levels at once and you develop indigestion, then it will be more difficult to identify the culprit. I know that garlic gives me indigestion. Because I have added supplements slowly over the years, it was easy for me to identify garlic as my culprit.

Be careful with supplement brand choice. Neither the cheapest nor the most expensive is necessarily the best. The most important thing is to buy reliable, quality brands and to review the contents of the brands you choose. My website at www.healthyjointsforlife.com may be helpful in choosing reliable supplements.

Supplements, like all foods and nutrients, are broken down by the body at different rates. We know, for example, that curcumin is metabolized quickly, so that is why I recommend taking it more frequently—two times a day. Fat soluble vitamins, like vitamin D, tend to be metabolized more slowly, so they don't need to be taken as frequently—one time a day. Space out your supplements, taking some in the morning and some in the evening, so they are more likely to be bioavailable to the body when needed.

LEVEL I	
SUPPLEMENT	RECOMMENDED DAILY DOSAGE
Vitamin C	500 mg 2x/day
Vitamin D$_3$	2000–5000 IU 1x/day
Vitamin E total mixed	100 IU 1x/day
Vitamin E gamma-tocotrienol	15 mg 1x/day
Calcium	250 mg 2x/day
Omega-3s	1000 mg 2x/day
Green tea	270 mg total EGCG in 2–3 separate doses
Glucosamine	1500 mg 1x/day
Chondroitin	1200 mg 1x/day
Silymarin	200 mg 2x/day

MOVE

STARTING SLOWLY

This week you will be implementing your customized aerobic, flexibility, and resistance exercise plan. You get to decide which exercises you will do (choosing from those presented in Chapter 5), and I will tell you how many days a week to exercise and how much time to spend on each session. Remember, you need to do only the exercises you can tolerate; choose based on your experience and relative joint health.

As Chapter 5 notes, the amount of exercise you do will be based on the degree of joint disease that you have. Additionally, the joints that are affected will determine which exercises are possible for you. For instance, if your shoulder hurts, don't overdo shoulder exercises. But if your knees feel great, go ahead and pursue any and all exercises involving the knees. If you are reading this book, it is most likely that your joints are really bothering you, so I'm introducing you to exercise very slowly. The time frames of this plan were deliberately developed for those of you with the most severe disease. If you are already in good shape and are suffering from relatively little pain, then start with the duration and frequency of exercise outlined for subsequent weeks, maybe even weeks six, seven, or eight. I don't want to hold anyone back!

Use Chapter 5 as your guide, and pick and choose from the offered activities for each of the exercise categories listed below. Remember that both resistance exercises and flexibility exercises can be done to accommodate your level of pain or flexibility. If you have severe knee pain, then choose resistance exercises from the "severe" part of the resistance exercise menu (isometrics). If you have mild shoulder pain, then choose resistance exercises from the "mild" part of the menu (weight training). If you are not sure which resistance exercises to do, start with the less aggressive "severe" pain resistance exercises. You can always work your way up. Don't get discouraged by biting off more than you can chew. It's not where you start, but where you finish, and I want you to ease into exercise so you can finish strong and make exercise a part of your new joint-healthy life!

EXERCISE ACTIVITIES

Aerobic	5 minutes	2x/week
Flexibility	5 minutes	2x/week
Resistance	10 minutes	2x/week

WEEK 1 SAMPLE SCHEDULE

Monday	5 minutes warm-up and flexibility 5 minutes aerobic 10 minutes resistance
Tuesday	Rest
Wednesday	Rest
Thursday	Rest
Friday	5 minutes warm-up and flexibility 5 minutes aerobic 10 minutes resistance
Saturday	Rest
Sunday	Rest

CHAPTER 8

WEEK TWO:
Healthy Joints for Life

EAT

ADDING FIBER

YOUR PANTRY AND FRIDGE SHOULD STILL BE JOINT FRIENDLY, AND your six meals and snacks schedule should be established. Each subsequent week we are going to fine-tune your diet to get you to joint health. The dietary focus of this week is adding fiber to your diet—particularly in snacks—to increase your feeling of fullness and help you bridge the gap between meals.

Most people don't get enough fiber, so make a conscious effort to add fiber-rich foods to your diet. Another easy way to do this is by putting fiber powder in water or a smoothie and consuming it as a snack. Various manufacturers offer fiber powders in different flavors. Experiment with types and flavors to find one that works for you. Despite their reputations they actually taste fine. My favorite fiber drink is what I call a Fiber Creamsicle Smoothie (see recipe below). Try it, especially if you have a sweet tooth. If drinks or smoothies aren't appealing to you, then you could also get your fiber in tablet form (Fiber Choice) or even gummy form (Vitafusion Fiber Gummies).

FIBER CREAMSICLE SMOOTHIE RECIPE

1 teaspoon orange-flavored Metamucil

1 tablespoon sugar-free yogurt

½ scoop (⅛ cup) vanilla protein powder

3–4 ice cubes

1 cup water

Combine all the ingredients in a blender and blend until smooth.

Your goal is to consume a total of twenty to twenty-five grams of fiber daily. Some fiber will come from your smoothies, shakes, or tablets. The rest should come from your diet. Don't shortchange yourself when it comes to your diet. Make sure that you get at least ten grams of fiber from whole foods. See pages 46–48 for a listing of fiber-rich foods.

MEAL SCHEDULE	
8:00 a.m.–9:00 a.m.	Breakfast (soluble and insoluble fiber from food)
Midmorning	Snack (opportunity to include fiber)
12:00 p.m.–1:00 p.m.	Lunch (soluble and insoluble fiber from food)
3:00 p.m.	Snack (opportunity to include fiber)
6:00 p.m.–7:00 p.m.	Dinner (soluble and insoluble fiber from food)
8:00 p.m.–9:00 p.m.	Snack (opportunity to include fiber)

SUPPLEMENT

STEADY ON COURSE

Continue with Level I supplements this week.

MOVE

SLOWLY LUBRICATING JOINTS

In the first week you exercised only two times. Forty minutes in a whole week! This is intentional, a slow and sure way to get you started. Continue on this gentle schedule and gradually introduce exercise to those achy joints. We don't want to overwhelm you or your joints. For those of you with less pain and arthritic disease, feel free to jump ahead to subsequent weeks.

In week two maintain your exercise routine and be sure you are choosing the exercises that are suited to your intensity level of joint pain or disease. If you are having trouble with any aspect of exercise, try doing a combination of exercises (e.g., biking and walking), doing fewer reps, or decreasing your time spent exercising. Most of you should be doing fine with this light introduction to moving. If you are exceeding my expectations and doing the exercises with ease, try increasing the number of reps or your time spent working out. You can always make adjustments to the frequency and intensity of your exercise workouts.

EXERCISE ACTIVITIES		
Aerobic	5 minutes	2x/week
Flexibility	5 minutes	2x/week
Resistance	10 minutes	2x/week

WEEK 2 SAMPLE SCHEDULE	
Monday	5 minutes warm-up and flexibility 5 minutes aerobic 10 minutes resistance
Tuesday	Rest
Wednesday	Rest
Thursday	Rest
Friday	5 minutes warm-up and flexibility 5 minutes aerobic 10 minutes resistance
Saturday	Rest
Sunday	Rest

CHAPTER 9

WEEK THREE:
Healthy Joints for Life

EAT

INTRODUCING VARIOUS PROTEIN SOURCES

IN THIS WEEK, PUTTING THE PROPER PROTEIN, SUCH AS SALMON, other seafood, and lean meats, on your plate will yield great results. Vary the protein sources each day to achieve the maximum benefit and to avoid falling into a dietary rut.

Now it is time to think about the amount of protein you consume, as well as the protein sources you select. Remember, protein is good, but some sources of protein also have bad saturated fats, which is not so good.

Try to eat wild Alaskan sockeye salmon at least two times a week. Substitute another fish if you don't like salmon. Try to eat a crustacean (crab, lobster, shrimp) at least once a week. This will get you eating seafood three times per week. Obviously, if you don't (vegetarian), won't ("Yuck! I hate the taste!"), or can't (allergic) eat seafood, then throw that suggestion out the door and substitute in the other joint-healthy protein choices we've discussed, like chicken, turkey, buffalo, grass-fed beef, and pork. For those of you with fish or shellfish allergies, take omega-3s in supplement form. Omega XL brand (www.omegaxl.com) is said to be free of allergens so that people with shellfish allergies can use it. Pure, burpless and odorless omega-3s are available and highly recommended.

If you are a vegetarian, you'll need to get your protein elsewhere. Eat green veggies with a low GI, like spinach and kale. Spinach packs a 1:1 protein to carbohydrate ratio, whereas kale has a 1:3 ratio. Spinach wins as a protein source, but kale has a higher ORAC (approximately 1800 versus 1500). The beans and lentils recommended in Chapter 3 can also supply significant protein. Kidney beans offer one gram of protein for every one gram of carbohydrate, whereas lentils provide one gram of protein for every one gram of digestible carbohydrate and one gram of fiber. Various nut butters supply some protein at a modest carb load. Almond butter and peanut butter are probably best. The ratio of protein to carbohydrate to fiber for almond butter is 4:6:1, whereas the same ratio for peanut butter is about 4:2:1. Peanut butter is, therefore, better, but beware of its caloric density. Eat too much nut butter and you will gain weight. Tofu, a soy product, is a staple of most vegetarian diets. It is joint healthy, with an approximate 4:1 ratio of protein to carbohydrate and a very limited saturated fat profile. Tempeh is also a soybean product. It is protein dense, with one cup providing as much protein as a buffalo burger, thirty grams. It has a protein to carbohydrate ratio of 2:1, and thus it obviously packs more carbs than a similar amount of tofu.

Protein powders, including hemp, for smoothies can be helpful for those who don't eat dairy. (Note that whey and casein protein powders are both derived from milk.) Quinoa is another popular source of protein for vegetarians, but its protein to carbohydrate ratio is an unfavorable 1:4. It does contain some fiber and has a lower GI of 53. In moderation it is a reasonable source of protein for vegetarians.

Soy milk and almond milk can provide protein, as well, and both have about a 1:2 protein to carbohydrate ratio. Soy milk is roughly two and a half times more caloric than almond milk, however. The sprouted breads I introduced in Chapter 3 can be used as a protein source, too. The makeup of sprouted breads is variable, so estimates of their protein to carbohydrate ratio are best determined by consulting the label. Remember to be careful of bread's glycemic load.

The number of grams of protein you eat needs to be equal to or greater than your weight in pounds. If you weigh two hundred pounds, then you should be eating two hundred grams of protein over the course of the day. Because dinner is usually the largest meal of the day, it can provide the largest proportion of protein in your diet, but breakfast (eggs), snacks (yogurt, cottage cheese), and lunch (sliced meats) can also supply large amounts of protein and shouldn't be ignored as opportunities to eat protein.

You may prefer a larger lunch and a smaller dinner or the opposite. Maybe your family enjoys eating a big breakfast together. Try salmon in the form of lox with your breakfast and have your grass-fed beef (steak) with eggs. How you do it is up to you, but I want to introduce variety into your diet in order for you to get all those special nutrients those different foods offer.

In the protein schedule below there is nothing special about the specific days of the week that I have assigned to different protein sources. I have deliberately tried to keep things fresh by varying protein sources. I don't want your menus to become monotonous, but if you have a favorite, you certainly could eat it on consecutive days.

PROTEIN THROUGHOUT THE WEEK	
Monday	Fish (grilled)
Tuesday	Chicken (sautéed)
Wednesday	Grass-fed beef (grilled)

continued

PROTEIN THROUGHOUT THE WEEK	
Thursday	Fish (panfried)
Friday	Pork (baked)
Saturday	Crustacean (broiled, boiled, baked, or grilled)
Sunday	Turkey (roasted)

SUPPLEMENT

ADDING LEVEL II SUPPLEMENTS— ASSESSING TOLERANCE

Add Level II supplements to Level I supplements this week.

LEVEL II	
SUPPLEMENT	RECOMMENDED DAILY DOSAGE
Lutein	10–40 mg 1x/day
Astaxanthin	2–4 mg 1x/day
Vitamin B_6	10–20 mg 1x/day
Vitamin B total mixed	Multi of B_1–B_{12} 1x/day
PAC/Grape seed extract	200 mg 2x/day
Pomegranate extract	250–500 mg 2x/day
Ginger	500–1000 mg 1x/day

MOVE

SLOWLY GETTING UP TO SPEED

The amount of strength training increases this week to put some more power in your workout. As you increase your aerobic activity, you may choose to cross-train, intermingling activities like walking and biking or swimming and doing the elliptical machine. Alternatively, if you've found that swimming is just the perfect aerobic exercise for your joints, then simply do it for a longer period of time, as prescribed below. As you increase your resistance training, you will be adding to either the number of repetitions or the number of sets. Remember, in the beginning you may not be able to accomplish all the exercises in the prescribed time. Be patient, because as the program expands, there will be additional time to do more.

EXERCISE ACTIVITIES		
Aerobic	10 minutes	2x/week
Flexibility	5 minutes	3x/week
Resistance	15 minutes	2x/week

WEEK 3 SAMPLE SCHEDULE	
Monday	5 minutes warm-up and flexibility 10 minutes aerobic 15 minutes resistance
Tuesday	Rest
Wednesday	5 minutes warm-up and flexibility
Thursday	Rest
Friday	5 minutes warm-up and flexibility 10 minutes aerobic 15 minutes resistance
Saturday	Rest
Sunday	Rest

CHAPTER 10

WEEK FOUR:
Healthy Joints for Life

EAT

RESTRICTING CARBS

AT WEEK FOUR RESTRICT CARBOHYDRATES TO NO MORE THAN fifty grams per day. Although fiber is technically a carb, you don't need to count fiber as a carb in your daily carb totals, because it can't be digested like other carbs and doesn't affect insulin. Eat a vegetable with a different bright color at lunch and dinner. Step outside your comfort zone and try some kale or spicy peppers. Don't allow your carbs in any one meal to be greater than about twenty to twenty-five grams, and as mentioned above, the total for the entire day must be below fifty grams. See www.healthyjointsforlife.com for a more detailed carb counter. Carb-counting booklets by Drs. Atkins, Heller, or Eades could be helpful (see resources).

SUGGESTED PROTEIN AND VEGETABLE COMBINATIONS	
Monday	Grilled fish with grilled zucchini drizzled with olive oil
Tuesday	Chicken sautéed with kale, broccoli rabe, or bok choy and garlic
Wednesday	Grilled grass-fed beef with tomatoes and onions/scallions sautéed in olive oil and mashed cauliflower
Thursday	Panfried fish with chickpea, lentil, and barley salad and baked yams
Friday	Roasted pork with baked and browned Brussels sprouts and mushrooms
Saturday	Broiled, boiled, baked, or grilled crustacean with baked or steamed broccoli drizzled with olive oil and lemon
Sunday	Ground buffalo meat sautéed with peppers and scallions and cole slaw with minimal carrots and light mayonnaise

SUPPLEMENT

MAINTAINING LEVEL I AND II SUPPLEMENTS

Continue with Level I and Level II supplements this week.

MOVE

MAKING EXERCISE MORE REGULAR

Increase your aerobic activity to three times per week to get your heart pumping and your joints moving. Be gentle. Remember, it's not where you start, but where you finish.

EXERCISE ACTIVITIES		
Aerobic	10 minutes	3x/week
Flexibility	5 minutes	3x/week
Resistance	15 minutes	2x/week

WEEK 4 SAMPLE SCHEDULE	
Monday	5 minutes warm-up and flexibility 10 minutes aerobic 15 minutes resistance
Tuesday	Rest
Wednesday	5 minutes warm-up and flexibility 10 minutes aerobic
Thursday	Rest
Friday	5 minutes warm-up and flexibility 10 minutes aerobic 15 minutes resistance
Saturday	Rest
Sunday	Rest

CHAPTER 11

WEEK FIVE:
Healthy Joints for Life

EAT

CONCENTRATING ON HEALTHY FATS

IT IS TIME TO FOCUS ON HEALTHY FATS TO HELP SLOW CARBO-hydrate absorption and curb insulin secretion, which in turn will reduce inflammation. Don't forget that healthy fats can be tasty. Add some delicious organic extra-virgin olive oil to your salad, a dollop of whipped cream to your fresh berries, a few sliced almonds to your asparagus, and guacamole or avocado slices to your turkey sandwich on thinly sliced sprouted bread.

Remember, fats are calorie dense. A gram of fat has nine calories, whereas a gram of protein or carbohydrate has only four. This tells you that handful after handful of almonds or pistachios can add up, contributing too many calories to your diet.

Because this is the week when we are stressing fat consumption, we need to seriously consider omega-6 versus omega-3 ratios. Your new pantry should preclude you from consuming too many omega-6s. But because omega-6s can derail your program, be sure you are reading labels so you don't get tricked into eating trans fats, too. I like olive oil in general, but with a smoke point of 375°F (the point at which the oil starts to break down and its by-products don't taste good), it's not the most stable for cooking at high temperatures. I recommend using refined coconut oil for cooking (it is only 2 percent omega-6 and has a smoke point of 450°F, as compared to virgin coconut oil, which has a smoke point of 350°F), but for those who dislike the taste of coconut, avocado oil (more expensive) has a similar composition to olive oil but a higher smoke point, 510°F. Therefore, it is an excellent substitute. Definitely avoid corn oil (58 percent omega-6), peanut oil (32 percent omega-6), sunflower oil (68 percent omega-6), and safflower oil (78 percent omega-6). Of the more common oils, canola oil is 22 percent omega-6, which is significantly more than olive oil (10 percent), avocado oil (10 percent), and coconut oil (2 percent), but much better than corn, peanut, sunflower, and safflower oil (for more information, see www.scientificpyschic.com/fitness/fattyacids1.htlm, www.olivado.com/studies4.htm, www.en.wikipedia.org/wiki/Smoke_point).

SUPPLEMENT

ADDING LEVEL III SUPPLEMENTS— ASSESSING TOLERANCE

Add Level III supplements to Level I and Level II supplements this week.

LEVEL III	
SUPPLEMENT	RECOMMENDED DAILY DOSAGE
Curcumin (biocurcumax)	250–500 mg 2x/day
NAC	600 mg 1x/day

MOVE

STARTING TO GAIN POWER

Your aerobic and flexibility workouts are of longer duration this week. So, too, is your resistance training. You will be increasing stamina while improving ligament flexibility. You will also be building muscle that will help stabilize your joints while facilitating smooth motion.

EXERCISE ACTIVITIES		
Aerobic	15 minutes	3x/week
Flexibility	10 minutes	3x/week
Resistance	20 minutes	2x/week

WEEK 5 SAMPLE SCHEDULE	
Monday	10 minutes warm-up and flexibility 15 minutes aerobic 20 minutes resistance
Tuesday	Rest
Wednesday	10 minutes warm-up and flexibility 15 minutes aerobic

continued

WEEK 5 SAMPLE SCHEDULE	
Thursday	Rest
Friday	10 minutes warm-up and flexibility 15 minutes aerobic 20 minutes resistance
Saturday	Rest
Sunday	Rest

CHAPTER 12

WEEK SIX:
Healthy Joints for Life

EAT

MAINTAINING GROWTH HORMONE SECRETION

DURING THE NIGHT, WHILE WE SLEEP, THE BODY GOES INTO starvation mode. The unfortunate consequence of starvation mode is that growth hormone secretion is stunted. During this week, eat a slow-digesting casein protein shake or bar within an hour of bedtime to try to keep your body out of starvation mode. Casein is one of the two forms of protein derived from milk, whey being the other. Whey is quickly absorbed by the body, whereas casein is slowly absorbed. You can take advantage of casein's slow absorption characteristic to keep yourself out of starvation mode while you are sleeping. You can buy casein protein powder and make a shake by adding a scoop of protein powder (twenty-five grams of protein) to water and ice and blending it all together. Or buy a prepackaged casein protein shake or a casein protein bar.

Alternatively, you could opt for a recently developed SuperStarch shake before bed. Generation UCAN (GenerationUcan.com), a small

Connecticut-based company, developed the SuperStarch product as a treatment for patients with the metabolic inability to store sugars. It comes as a powder and can be mixed with water. The molecular makeup of SuperStarch renders it a slowly digested carb that doesn't bump insulin levels to the degree that regular carbs do. The size and complexity of the SuperStarch molecule makes it difficult for the body to digest quickly. This slow absorption works nicely with our program, keeping your body out of starvation mode.

Pre-bedtime eating is important because of its effect on growth hormone secretion, which peaks in the wee hours of the morning and is greater if you are not in starvation mode. As we age, growth hormone secretion decreases dramatically. Having an empty stomach during a night's sleep simulates starvation and further decreases growth hormone secretion. From a survival standpoint this makes sense. Would you be trying to "grow" or build muscle if you were starving? Of course not. You'd be trying to conserve your energy for survival, not muscle growth. The pre-bedtime eating technique is not so much an attempt to boost growth hormones as much as it is an effort to fight off the inevitable decline. Preserving growth hormone is important for muscle mass preservation and tendon strength and, therefore, our aging and aching joints!

SUPPLEMENT

FEELING THE BENEFITS
OF LEVEL III SUPPLEMENTS

Continue with Level I, Level II, and Level III supplements this week.

MOVE

GETTING MORE JOINT MOVEMENT AND LUBRICATION

You've now arrived at that twenty-minute mark of aerobic exercise, the ideal amount of time for lubrication production and joint strengthening. You are helping your joints, helping your heart, and reducing your risk for a litany of cancers. Be proud. Maintain variety and keep your workouts interesting. Swap walking for using a stationary bike. Take a break from the treadmill and try the rowing machine. Experiment as your body starts to respond to the stresses you are putting on it. Your muscles should be getting stronger and your flexibility should be improving.

EXERCISE ACTIVITIES		
Aerobic	20 minutes	3x/week
Flexibility	10 minutes	3x/week
Resistance	20 minutes	2x/week

WEEK 6 SAMPLE SCHEDULE	
Monday	10 minutes warm-up and flexibility 20 minutes aerobic 20 minutes resistance
Tuesday	Rest
Wednesday	10 minutes warm-up and flexibility 20 minutes aerobic
Thursday	Rest

continued

WEEK 6 SAMPLE SCHEDULE	
Friday	10 minutes warm-up and flexibility 20 minutes aerobic 20 minutes resistance
Saturday	Rest
Sunday	Rest

CHAPTER 13

WEEK SEVEN:
Healthy Joints for Life

EAT

WATCHING CALORIES

NOW THAT YOU HAVE ESTABLISHED GOOD EATING HABITS, IT IS time to pay closer attention to the calorie content of the individual foods you are eating and the cumulative calorie counts of your meals.

By now, the basic format for your dietary program should be established, but it's time to refine things. You have figured out how frequently you need to eat and have incorporated snacks between meals to curb uncontrolled hunger. You are eating healthy protein, carbs, and fats, concentrating on how they best work together. You've added in fiber with snacks for all their inherent benefits, as well as a bedtime snack to help prevent the decline in growth hormone secretion.

Carbs drive hunger. You have probably experienced this phenomenon yourself: eat high-carbohydrate Chinese food and two hours later you're starving for more. Usually, high-protein, low–refined carbohydrate diets help to curb hunger. It's the reason why the Atkins

Diet is easy to follow. Dr. Atkins said to eat whatever amount of protein you want, knowing that without carbs to trigger them, the brain's hunger centers would eventually be subdued.

This week you will start a food-and-drink journal to document exactly what you are eating and drinking and how much. Write down the calories and the grams of protein, carbs, and fat of everything that you eat throughout the day—snacks and beverages included. This is going to take an effort on your behalf, but if you've made it this far, I have confidence that you will be willing to make the effort to refine the way you eat and maximize the end result.

KEEPING A FOOD-AND-DRINK JOURNAL

Your food-and-drink journal can be kept any way that you prefer, in a spiral notebook, on your tablet, or in your phone—whatever is the easiest method for you to keep track of the foods and drinks you consume during the day. Write down what you are eating and drinking, along with their calories and grams of protein, carbs, and fat. Not only will this give you a big picture of what you are consuming throughout the day (and week), but it will also let you know if you are keeping these nutrients in balance. See the resources section for the handy pocket-size calorie, fat, protein, and carb counters. You may be surprised to learn how much or how little you are consuming. You don't have to keep the journal forever, just long enough so that you can evaluate what you are eating and drinking on a regular basis.

In most cases the *Healthy Joints for Life* diet program takes care of itself, but if your joint pain isn't going away, it is important to determine why. For the diet to work, you should be consuming reasonable portions and not overloading on bad fats or high-glycemic carbs. I've seen patients do some weird things that derail the diet. One patient put an exuberant amount of olive oil on his salad but then would drink the remaining olive oil from the bottom of the salad bowl. He was drinking about four tablespoons of olive oil from the bottom of the bowl each night, accounting for 480 extra calories a day. After eight weeks he hadn't lost a pound, and the olive oil alone represented about eight pounds of weight gain! Sometimes too much of a good thing can be detrimental, so keeping tabs on what you are consuming is important.

SUPPLEMENT

ADDING LEVEL IV SUPPLEMENTS— ASSESSING TOLERANCE

Add Level IV supplements to Level I, Level II, and Level III supplements this week.

LEVEL IV	
SUPPLEMENT	RECOMMENDED DAILY DOSAGE
Resveratrol	250 mg 1x/day
Boswellia	300 mg 2x/day
Licorice root* (maximum 1-month cycle)	400 mg of glycyrrhizic acid 1x/day (maximum dose)

*Note: If you have high blood pressure eliminate licorice root from your supplement program. Even patients with normal blood pressure should be careful with licorice root. Do not take licorice root daily for more than one month at a time because of possible blood pressure side effects. After taking it for one month, stay off it for one month. Do not take more than the recommended daily dosage for the active component of licorice root, glycyrrhizic acid.

MOVE

HITTING THE SWEET SPOT

This week's workouts remain at three times per week for aerobic and flexibility, and stay at two times per week for resistance. The only change is that resistance workouts increase to 25 minutes. All together it is still less than three hours a week for exercise.

EXERCISE ACTIVITIES		
Aerobic	20 minutes	3x/week
Flexibility	10 minutes	3x/week
Resistance	25 minutes	2x/week

WEEK 7 SAMPLE SCHEDULE	
Monday	10 minutes warm-up and flexibility 20 minutes aerobic 25 minutes resistance
Tuesday	Rest
Wednesday	10 minutes warm-up and flexibility 20 minutes aerobic
Thursday	Rest
Friday	10 minutes warm-up and flexibility 20 minutes aerobic 25 minutes resistance
Saturday	Rest
Sunday	Rest

CHAPTER 14

WEEK EIGHT:
Healthy Joints for Life

EAT

ASSESSING HYDRATION

THE PROGRAM SHOULD BE HUMMING ALONG QUITE NICELY AT this point. The last topic to discuss and incorporate into the program is water consumption. The human body is about 60 percent water. Since muscle contains 75 percent water and fat closer to 50 percent, it stands to reason that as you build muscle and drop fat, you will need more water. If you have been following the program, you have maintained or built muscle and decreased fat, so you need to adjust your hydration level.

We know that drinking water helps to preserve the health of your teeth, aids in digestion, and flushes out toxins. Your skin wrinkles with dehydration and glistens when hydrated. Your muscles cramp when dehydrated, and your joint cartilage becomes less rubbery and resilient as water content decreases. Water is important.

Good hydration is the perfect complement to any diet and workout program. Drinking water can help curb appetite and allow further weight reduction. You may already be hydrating sufficiently, but if you are not drinking enough water, you may be missing out on the obvious benefits of sufficient water consumption. Each cell in your body is like a mini ocean, with nutrients carried in the sea of life. Dehydration negatively effects cell function, resulting in suboptimal cell performance. That may manifest itself as a lack of energy and strength or as dizziness and a lack of mental acuity. Your brain doesn't work well without water. Your muscles don't contract normally without water, and your joints don't cushion as well without water.

The minimum daily consumption of water is about seventy-two ounces, a little more if you are bigger and a little less if you are smaller. Consuming that amount should be easily accomplished by drinking twelve ounces with breakfast, twelve ounces between breakfast and lunch, twelve ounces at lunch, twelve ounces between lunch and dinner, twelve ounces at dinner, and twelve ounces with your bedtime protein or SuperStarch drink. If your nighttime snack/dessert is a hot chocolate or a cup of green tea, then you can count that as your last round of water, or drink the water, anyway. It can't hurt. Remember, there is water in mangosteen juice, tea, hot chocolate, seltzer, and calorie-free flavored waters. Staying hydrated is important for controlling hunger, as well as for increasing your body's metabolism.

Consider this: When you drink cold water, your body temperature decreases. Your body will then increase your metabolism ever so slightly to get your core temperature to 98.6 degrees. So just by drinking cold water, you are helping your metabolism, even if only slightly.

Joint cartilage is largely water, and as we age, the water content in our joints decreases. That means both cushioning and lubrication decrease. Drinking some water won't immediately restore the water content of cartilage. However, chronic dehydration might contribute to this reduction in the water content of joints. Stay hydrated!

SUPPLEMENT

FULLY IMPLEMENTED

Continue with Level I, Level II, Level III, and Level IV supplements this week.

MOVE

EXERCISING FOR LIFE

Your exercise habits should be well established, and you can continue with this final week's program as your permanent exercise regimen. You will note that resistance training is increased to 30 minutes. Remember that you can vary your workouts by increasing or decreasing your intensity or time. Try a little longer workout if you feel great, and spend a little less time, rather than skipping a workout, if time is short. Some days may be leisurely, and others more intense. Change up the activities you do, swimming one day and biking another, for instance. Don't do the same strength training every week. Pick different exercises off the menu from Chapter 5. Switching venues from your home gym to your friend's gym or exercising outside may add a breath of fresh air to your workouts. Workouts don't have to be sterile or strictly "by the book." Try a yoga class or get involved in water aerobic classes. Do some Zumba or take an invigorating step class. Try a new DVD. Don't be afraid to challenge yourself, but don't push yourself so hard that you don't want to (or can't) move the next day. Understand but don't dwell on your limitations. Don't overreach your ability and get hurt. Never let exercise become an albatross, a burden. It is important to understand that this program is to help improve your life, not be your life. Keep a positive attitude, keep your goals in mind, and look forward, not backward. Exercise in a way that is pleasant and refreshing and rejuvenating.

EXERCISE ACTIVITIES		
Aerobic	20 minutes	3x/week
Flexibility	10 minutes	3x/week
Resistance	30 minutes	2x/week

WEEK 8 SAMPLE SCHEDULE	
Monday	10 minutes warm-up and flexibility 20 minutes aerobic 30 minutes resistance
Tuesday	Rest
Wednesday	10 minutes warm-up and flexibility 20 minutes aerobic
Thursday	Rest
Friday	10 minutes warm-up and flexibility 20 minutes aerobic 30 minutes resistance
Saturday	Rest
Sunday	Rest

***

Congratulations! You have made it through all the basic science surrounding joint pain, the science behind the natural remedies, and the implementation of the program—all in eight weeks! You've learned about things you probably never imagined you would or thought you could. You now have the knowledge to succeed. As much progress as you have made at this point, you will keep improving as time goes on. Keep it up and you will continue to strengthen your muscles and ligaments. Your joint lubrication will continue to improve, inflammation will lessen, and your joint pain will diminish. You should be feeling lighter and more flexible, experiencing less pain, and finding yourself able to participate in more of the amazing things that life has to offer. Taking control of your joint pain is freeing you from the imprisonment of joint pain. It's time to embrace life more fully. Get out there with your family and friends and see and enjoy the world.

I hope that you are convinced that it is time to be joint-healthy and heart healthy and cancer preventative. Pour yourself a few delicious ounces of mangosteen juice and chase down a handful of my recommended joint-healthy supplements. Enjoy a delicious piece of olive oil–rubbed roasted chicken sprinkled with rosemary and thyme. Doesn't it feel great to know that you're helping your painful joints while taking premium care of your heart and reducing your cancer risk?

There's no better time than now to start your new lifestyle. Don't make excuses; it's time to help yourself. You have the knowledge to make it all happen. You now know that diet, exercise, and supplements can deliver you to joint health and more. As a youngster, I would practice playing football in the front yard with my dad. Sometimes I played well, and other times not so well. My dad always said the same thing when we finished. "Try your best and I'll always be proud of you." Before football games my dad used to whisper to me, "Make me proud." I knew exactly what that meant: he wanted my best effort, and with that he knew there would be success. Each time I heard those words, they became more powerful. They became a crucial part of my pregame ritual and pushed me to do my best. I fed off the fact that my dad, my family, and my friends were watching me, pulling for me, and hoping for me to succeed. I know that there are people all around you who are rooting for you to succeed.

I hope my words and this book can motivate you to make that crucial step forward to help yourself. You have my best wishes for a joint-healthy life. "Make me proud."

APPENDIX I

The Cell Science Behind It All

BECAUSE I AM AT HEART A MOLECULAR SCIENTIST, OR, AS THE young daughter of one of my patients put it, a molecular wizard, I love the details of how cells work. In order for you to gain a better understanding of the unique perspective that substantiates my program, in the previous pages I threw a fair amount of science at you. For some, the science may have been frustrating. For others, it may not have been enough. To get to the heart of the matter, I glossed over much of the heavyweight science, saving it for now, when you can dwell on the science as you wish, and I can live my passion in explaining it to you.

Let's start simply. The cell is a small enclosure that encapsulates even smaller structures. In many ways it is like a microscopic burlap sack. The outside wall of the sack is called the cell membrane. I compare the cell's membrane to burlap because, like burlap, the membrane is coarse and porous.

The membrane is primarily made of fat. Studding the fatty cell membrane are proteins, sugar/protein combination molecules, and cholesterol. A cell without cholesterol would be limp. Because the membrane is predominantly fat, a cell without fat would be like stew without a bowl—meat, carrots, peas, and gravy running all over the place. Fats serve as the building blocks for establishing a supple, flowing, dynamic compartment to contain and maintain the cell contents. Cholesterol adds some rigidity to the compartment. What you eat influences the fats that reside in your cell membranes, as so nicely shown by Neelands (1983), Vidgren (1997), Cao (2006), and Arterburn (2006).

THE CONTENTS OF THE CELL

The inside of the cell is like the contents of an extremely organized pot of stew. There is a fluidlike gravy called cytoplasm, which contains all the water, proteins, sodium, potassium, calcium, and other ions and nutrients that the cell and its contents need to function.

Floating in the "cytoplasmic gravy" are microscopic organelles. Organelle is the medical term for a "miniature organ." These organelles are like the peas, carrots, potatoes, and meat of the stew.

Organelles have different functions and are separated from one another by their own burlap, or membranes, but they are intrinsically interrelated, communicating with one another in order to enable the entire cell to function. Because they're wrapped in their own individual membrane, they can segregate their own enzymes and nutrients from one another so they can function without interrupting one another.

If you work with coworkers in the same room but at separate desks, you can relate to how the cell works. Each worker has his or her own desk with special supplies, like telephones, computers, and fax machines. A person with a different job may be assigned to each desk, the contents of each desk facilitating work on that assignment. The cell and its organelles are quite similar. And like your office, most of the time cellular activity works efficiently. However, sometimes small issues arise and trouble ensues. That's what happens when a cell is overwhelmed with inflammation.

COMMUNICATION THROUGH THE LOCK-AND-KEY MECHANISM

By unraveling and understanding the cell communication process that leads to inflammation, we can try to modify the process to our benefit.

Proteins and protein-sugars (glycoproteins) are important to cell membrane function and communication because they both guard and form channels through which molecules enter and exit the cell. Those channels are selective in allowing molecules in and out based on several features including ion or molecule size, charge, and shape. When molecular shape determines passage, the lock and key theory of molecular transport applies. The molecule serves as the key while the channel serves as the lock. When matching molecular "keys" fit into membrane "locks" (called receptors) travel through the membrane is allowed.

This lock-and-key mechanism is vitally important for transport and determination of what is inside the cell and what is outside the cell. Messenger molecules can only affect the function of a cell if they are allowed into the cell. The actual composition of the membrane is important too because the membrane does more than just serve as a barrier for compartmentalizing the cell. The membrane also supplies the individual membrane fats that are used to make many messenger molecules. Just like bricks are individual components of a brick wall, the fats of the membrane become the individual components of the messenger molecule. Use brownish-red bricks and you construct a brownish-red wall. Use healthy omega-3 fats and you construct anti-inflammatory messenger molecules.

If we can control what molecular messengers are produced, and how efficiently and effectively these molecules enter and exit the cell, we can influence what is being communicated. Let's start simple with an example. We know that "good" fats like omega-3s end up being "good" anti-inflammatory molecular messengers. We also know that when good fats populate the cell membrane, the fluidity of the membrane is better, allowing more efficient movement of molecules within and through the membrane. "Bad" fats do just the opposite, eventually becoming "bad" inflammatory molecular messengers and stiffening the cell membrane, making the appropriate flow of molecular messengers more difficult. Understanding and differentiating between which fats are good and which fats are bad will help you to decide which fats to eat.

YOU ARE WHAT YOU EAT?

It's true: you really are what you eat. The cells that currently make up your skin are not the same as the cells that made up your skin six months ago. Your skin is nearly brand-new every six months. Similarly, the miniature parts that make up the cells are changed regularly. This means, for example, that the cell membrane is repaired, rejuvenated, and replaced regularly. The fats that you eat go on to become the fats of the cell membrane. Neelands (1983), Cao (2006), Vidgren (1997), and Arterburn (2006) prove the concept that cell membrane structure and receptor function are directly affected by diet. Participants in these studies were specifically fed different-fat diets (saturated versus unsaturated) and then their cell membranes were analyzed for the content of those fats. It was shown that the type of fat consumption directly affected membrane composition. Eat more saturated fats and your cell membranes end up containing more saturated fats. Eat more unsaturated fats and your cell membranes contain more unsaturated fats. This is important because it provides scientific proof that we can alter the composition of our cell membranes away from inflammatory fats and toward anti-inflammatory fats.

What you eat becomes what your cell membranes are made of. This ground-breaking research proves that it is possible to influence cellular composition and function through diet.

THE LIPID BILAYER

The cell membrane fats are arranged in a bilayer. Bilayer literally means "two layers," so two layers of fat are stacked on top of one another. I like to think of it as a sandwich, with the bread representing the two layers, while my wife thinks the bilayer resembles a delicious double-layer chocolate cake. This less delicious diagram shows a magnification of a portion of the cell membrane bilayer.

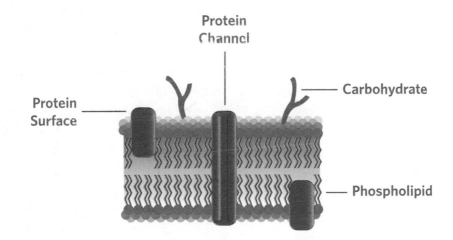

The membrane functions by allowing certain things into the cell while keeping certain things out. To accomplish this, each cell membrane layer is made up of a fat-soluble "fatty-acid tail" connected to a water-soluble "phosphate head," as shown in the following diagram.

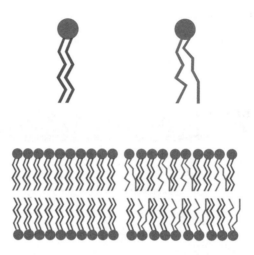

The layers are not stacked randomly. The phosphate groups (round heads) form the innermost and outermost aspects, while the fatty-acid tails (jagged lines) abut one another internally. This gives the bilayer two water-soluble areas (where the round heads are located) and a large fat-soluble internal area (where the jagged lines are located). To better understand how this works, watching animation videos on the internet can prove extremely worthwhile. Seeing 3 dimensional depictions can make these concepts come to life. (Go to youtube.com/watch?feature=fvwp&NR=1&v=Rl5EmUQdkuI and youtube.com/watch?v=S7-VFJHd0uA to watch two informative and educational introductions to the plasma membrane.)

Because fats are also called lipids and the fat is combined with a phosphate group, the basic building-block molecule of the bilayer is called a phospholipid. The bilayer's composition must be fluid enough to allow molecules to travel within, or across the membrane. The bilayer's fluidity can be altered by varying the type of fatty-acid tails. Some fatty-acid tails are stiff, while others are more pliable.

Membrane fluidity is determined by whether each one of the tails is shorter, longer, straight, or bent. This is important because we influence the shape of these fatty-acid tails by the fats that we eat.

DEFINING THE TYPES OF FATS
IN THE CELL MEMBRANE

Phospholipids are the primary building block of the cell membrane, and their fatty-acid tails are where the terms saturated and unsaturated come into play. I know the terms *saturated, unsaturated, monounsaturated* and *polyunsaturated* can be mind-boggling. I'm guessing you're hard-pressed to accurately define fat (though you know it on a steak), never mind saturated or unsaturated. Luckily, defining these terms isn't as complicated as it seems.

Fats are specific combinations of carbon, oxygen, and hydrogen. How they are combined determines saturation. Saturation is a function of bonds between two atoms. Carbon is an atom that is "satisfied" only if it forms four bonds or four connections. Carbon can bond to other substances, such as hydrogen or oxygen, or to other carbon atoms. Carbon binds with carbon at different levels of intensity. Two carbon atoms held together by a double bond are attached with roughly twice the intensity as a single bond. A single bond is, therefore, roughly half as strong as a double bond. A single bond fulfills one of the four bond requirements for the carbon atom, while a double bond fulfills two of the requirements.

Bonds are key in defining the terms *saturated* and *unsaturated*. *Saturated* means that the carbon atoms are connected by single bonds and have the maximum number of hydrogen atoms around them. (Remember that each carbon has to have a total of four bonds.) *Unsaturated* means that some carbon atoms are connected by double bonds. Each double bond satisfies two of the four bonds required per carbon atom. A carbon atom with a double bond has less than the maximum number of hydrogen atoms.

Monounsaturated means that a fat has one double bond, while *polyunsaturated* means that the fat has more than one double bond. In omega-3 fatty acids, the first double bond extends between carbon atom number three and carbon atom number four. Omega-6 fatty acids have the first double bond between carbon atom number six and carbon atom number seven. The name and number simply denote the location of the double bond.

These two particular fatty acids, omega-3 and omega-6, are called "essential" because humans do not have the enzymes that can produce them. Therefore, we have to eat them, or we will become deficient. There are numerous types of omega-3 and omega-6 fatty acids. For example, DHA (docosahexanoic acid) and EPA (eicosapentanoic acid) are both very important omega-3s that we want to consume for joint health. They both have the same double bond at the 3 position but they are different in overall carbon length (22 carbons vs 20 carbons) and number of other double bonds (6 vs 5). This is a good example of how our nomenclature (how we name molecules) does not mention all double bonds, only the key third for omega-3s and the key sixth for omega-6s. If you are curious, linoleic acid (carbons-18, 2 double bonds) and arachidonic acid (carbons-20, 4 double bonds) are examples of common omega-6s and how they differ. Arachidonic acid is the omega-6 fatty acid that we particularly want to keep out of our cell membranes because it is a building block for inflammatory messengers.

WHY ARE SATURATED AND UNSATURATED FATS SO IMPORTANT FOR CELL MEMBRANE FUNCTION?

Saturated and unsaturated fats are important because of the shape imparted by the different bonds. Saturated fats impart a straight shape to the fatty-acid tail, while unsaturated fatty-acid tails are bent or crooked. The shapes can be helpful or detrimental to the stacking of the cell membrane.

The straight-shaped saturated fats stack up next to one another very closely, while the bent-shaped unsaturated fats can't stack up as closely. A lipid bilayer with some unsaturated fats makes the cell membrane more porous. Just like it's difficult to walk down a crowded New York City street, it's tough to travel through a densely packed membrane composed solely of saturated fats. A cell membrane with a mixture of fats is like an uncongested sidewalk: it's easier for molecules to "walk" from one place to another.

SATURATED AND UNSATURATED FATS
DO MORE THAN MAKE UP THE CELL MEMBRANE

The saturated and unsaturated fats you eat make up a large portion of the lipid bilayer. In the cell membrane they have a dual role. They help establish stiffness or fluidity, and they also become the building blocks for the cellular production of pro- or anti-inflammatory messengers. Cholesterol, which many people mistake for a fat, is not a fat, but a sterol (cholesterol). Cholesterol is a precursor or building-block molecule for steroid hormones, like testosterone and estrogen. It is also an essential component of the cell membrane.

Too much cholesterol and the cell membrane becomes too rigid. Too much saturated fat and the cell membrane becomes too firmly packed. With the right amount of cholesterol and saturated and unsaturated fats, you have a fluid, communicative cell membrane.

For joint health, it's important to understand that omega-6 fats in the cell membrane can be plucked out of the membrane and processed into inflammatory messengers, while omega-3 cell membrane fats become anti-inflammatory messengers. The more omega-6 fats there are in the cell membrane, the larger the potential for inflammatory-molecule production. We are desperately trying to avoid the accumulation of omega-6 fats in the cell membrane (Hwang 1997).

THE NUCLEUS—
THE CELL'S CONTROL CENTER

The nucleus is the cell's brains—its control center. It is a membrane-enclosed sac of genetic material called DNA—deoxyribonucleic acid.

DNA comes in the shape of a twisted ladder, referred to scientifically as a double helix. This double helix creates an extraordinarily reliable system of protein production that directs the cell. The DNA of each cell contains the codes or templates for tens of thousands of protein molecules, which, when appropriately produced, allow the cell, organ, and body to communicate and work seamlessly. Proteins are the cell messengers. How does the cell know which molecules to produce, in what quantity, and at what time? This represents part of the key to controlling inflammation. The rungs of the DNA ladder are matching interdigitating molecules called nucleotide pairs. Every three rungs on the ladder represent a code for an amino acid. A series of amino acids linked together forms a protein.

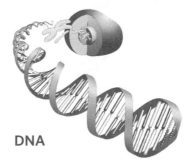

DNA

John M. Havel Illustration

There are three billion rungs on the DNA ladder. These rungs collectively form your genes. They determine your eye, hair, and skin color. They code for your hormones and all the proteins that regulate your bodily functions. Because of the staggering amount of information coded in these three billion rungs, it is vital that the DNA knows what portion is on and what portion is off. A precise and efficient system must exist to produce the correct proteins for the appropriate situation. For example, if a protein needs to be made—let's say the COX-2 protein/enzyme, essential for the production of inflammatory molecules—the system must specifically identify the area of DNA where the COX-2 protein/enzyme is coded. There may be one million potential areas along the length of the DNA where distinctly different proteins are made. In this example, the COX-2 DNA site must be found quickly.

A DNA transcription factor, or "caretaker," as I like to refer to them, has the ability to locate a specific protein sequence to turn it on. NFkB, for example, by virtue of its three-dimensional shape, has the ability to locate the start sequence for innumerable inflammatory molecules, including COX-2. When the cell determines a protein is to be made, a specific process occurs. A particular DNA caretaker, with matching lock and key shapes, will activate a portion of the DNA. The DNA ladder unwinds and splits into a left half and a right half. Half the ladder acts as a template for a sequence of events that ultimately leads to the production of a protein that serves as a messenger molecule. Our job is to try to prevent the activation of DNA sequences where inflammatory proteins are made.

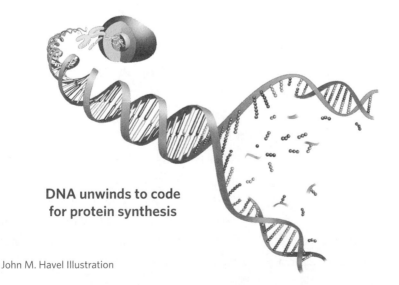

**DNA unwinds to code
for protein synthesis**

John M. Havel Illustration

UNDERSTANDING ENZYMES

An enzyme is a protein that speeds up a chemical reaction without being consumed or changed. Most enzymes speed up biological chemical reactions by one million!

THE INFLAMMATORY PATHWAYS

It's fascinating to trace the individual molecules of inflammation. There are pathways that increase inflammation, and there are those that stop inflammation.

Let's start with the most basic pathway of inflammation. The phospholipids that reside in the cell membrane can be metabolized or broken down by an enzyme called phospholipase A2. This enzyme separates the phosphate group from the fatty-acid group and converts the fatty acid into a very important molecule, arachidonic acid.

Let me give you an example of how this works. You decide to eat a store-bought salad dressing that seems healthy. You read the label and find it is made of soybean oil, a vegetable oil made of pro-inflammatory omega-6 fats. Through digestion, these omega-6 fatty acids from the salad dressing end up in millions of your cell membranes, ready to start the inflammatory cascade. If you had chosen olive oil instead of the salad dressing, you would not have supplied the omega-6 fatty acids that became arachidonic acid and you would not have ignited the inflammatory cascade (Bagga 2003).

Arachidonic acid is metabolized by the cyclooxygenase-2 enzyme (COX-2) into inflammatory prostaglandins (PG2s) or thromboxanes. If arachidonic acid is metabolized by lipoxygenase (LOX), another group of enzymes, called leukotrienes, is formed. PG2 prostaglandins call for inflammation, thromboxanes are part of the clotting cascade, and leukotrienes are responsible for airway constriction in asthma. All are part of the inflammatory process.

However, if omega-3 fatty acids are the membrane starting blocks, arachidonic acid isn't formed. Instead, the COX-2 enzyme will turn omega-3s into "good" prostaglandins (PG3s), which don't cause excessive inflammation (Fan 2004).

Just like there are "good" and "bad" cholesterols, there are "good" and "bad" prostaglandins. This is the big difference between consuming omega-6s and omega-3s.

HOW PAIN RELIEF WORKS

Aspirin, Advil, and Aleve, common over-the-counter anti-inflammatory medicines, work by blocking the COX-1 and COX-2 enzymes.

MODIFIED COX-2

In 2002 researcher Charles Serhan discovered that if omega-3 fatty acids are the starting blocks for a slightly modified COX-2 enzyme, resolvins and protectins are produced instead of prostaglandins. That modification, caused by taking a simple aspirin, adds a CH_3 group to the COX-2 enzyme—and makes a world of difference (Serhan 2004).

Just as the names imply, resolvins resolve inflammation and protectins protect from inflammation. Resolvins and protectins also decrease airway inflammation and protect nerve function, block white-blood-cell migration, and decrease the inflammatory molecular messengers tumor-necrosis-factor-alpha (TNF-alpha) and interferon-gamma (IFN-gamma).

Aspirin can have many positive effects on the body, including thinning the blood and, as mentioned above, modifying the COX-2 enzyme. If arachidonic acid is a starting block, the methylated (CH_3) COX-2 enzyme will produce epilipoxins, which are also anti-inflammatory.

Based on all this, it appears that an aspirin a day is better than an apple a day for keeping the orthopedic joint doctor away. Be careful, though, because aspirin is not without side effects. Aspirin is responsible for thousands of deaths yearly, because it can cause gastrointestinal bleeding. Larger doses are considered more risky, but even small doses (e.g., a baby aspirin) are associated with some risk. Closely related to aspirin, the nonsteroidal anti-inflammatories (NSAIDs), like over-the-counter Advil and Aleve, can also cause ulcers and adversely affect the kidneys.

The chart below summarizes the four chemical pathways you need to know. It's organized to show what you start with and what you end up with. It then states whether the end product is inflammatory or anti-inflammatory.

START WITH	ENZYME	END UP WITH	EFFECT
Arachidonic acid (from Omega-6 fatty acid)	•••••➤ COX-2 enzyme	Prostaglandin E2 (2 series)	Inflammatory
EPA, DHA (from Omega-3 fatty acid)	•••••➤ COX-2 enzyme	Prostaglandin E3 (3 series)	Anti-inflammatory
Arachidonic acid (from Omega-6 fatty acid)	•••••➤ Aspirin-modified COX-2 enzyme	Epilipoxin	Anti-inflammatory
EPA, DHA (from Omega-3 fatty acid)	•••••➤ Aspirin-modified COX-2 enzyme	Resolvins and Protectins	Anti-inflammatory

In case you didn't notice, *three out of the four* pathways are *anti-*inflammatory. However, there are two problems: There are many more omega-6 fatty acids to supply arachidonic acid than there are omega-3 fatty acids to provide EPA and DHA, and most of the individual COX-2 enzymes are not methylated. So, even though three of the four pathways are anti-inflammatory, the pathway doing the most is the one that causes inflammation—arachidonic acid becoming the "bad" prostaglandin E2.

We can curtail that pathway by doing three things:

1. Increase consumption of omega-3 fatty acids by eating more fish, like salmon or mackerel, or through supplementation.
2. Decrease consumption of omega-6 fatty acids by getting familiar with the foods that have an overabundance of omega-6s.
3. Take an aspirin a day to methylate the COX-2 enzymes, unless you have a history of stomach ulcers or your medical doctor advises otherwise.

INFLAMMATION, JOINT PAIN, OUR TOUGHEST OPPONENTS, AND MORE: THE REPRISE

I have to restate this information one last time: Joint pain is a problem involving several different cell types. There are bone cells called osteoblasts and osteoclasts, as well as different joint-lining cells and cartilage cells called chondrocytes. A variety of white blood cells also play a pivotal role in joint health. Each of these cells is on an inflammatory seesaw, being influenced by molecular messengers. Ultimately, these messengers cause cartilage degradation. These messengers are produced in response to various stimuli, both mechanical and molecular. Let's look at some of these more specifically.

There are several pro-inflammatory stimuli for articular cartilage degradation, including:

1. Stimulation of cartilage cell sensors called mechanoreceptors.
2. Stimulation of the cartilage cells via articular cartilage degradation products.
3. Interruption of the cartilage cell CD44 linkage.
4. Stimulation of the cartilage cells via free radicals.

Any or all of these stimuli can activate NFkB or other DNA caretakers located inside the cartilage cell, which leads to sinister inflammatory molecule production. Let's look at each of these processes more closely so you can understand them better.

STIMULATION OF CHONDROCYTE MECHANORECEPTORS

Mechanical stress can literally crack the articular cartilage through pressure caused by repeated impact or static compression of the joints. Smaller quantities of mechanical stress can also lead to problems when the stress activates specialized sensors, or mechanoreceptors, on cartilage cells that trigger the inflammatory process. Mechanoreceptors are sensitive and specialized receptors that have the ability to detect stress, much like your skin can feel the pressure of a landing mosquito. The types of stress that can trigger a response from chondrocyte mechanoreceptors vary from person to person, in the same way that people exhibit differences in their sensitivity to feeling a mosquito on their skin. What may initiate inflammation in one person may not affect another. The person with cells more sensitive to stress will, therefore, initiate inflammation more easily. That is perhaps one reason why one person laying carpet develops arthritic degeneration while another with the same job doesn't.

STIMULATION OF CHONDROCYTES VIA ARTICULAR CARTILAGE DEGRADATION PRODUCTS

When ECM breaks down, it stimulates cartilage cells, which leads to a further breakdown and damage to cartilage.

If you rub sandpaper against wood, you get sawdust. I like to think of the by-products of the overuse or abuse of cartilage, such as fibronectin fragments, as "cartilage sawdust." And just like sawdust in your eye can make it water, cartilage sawdust coming into contact with a cartilage cell or a cell of the synovium starts an inflammatory cascade—the process of secretion of battery acid–like, caustic inflammatory molecules called cytokines.

INTERRUPTION OF THE CHONDROCYTE CD44 LINKAGE

Using an electron microscope, the hyaluronan in cartilage matrix can be seen linking with receptors (CD44) on chondrocytes. This linkage keeps the chondrocytes happy. Interruption of the CD44-hyaluronan linkage leads to the activation of activator protein-1 (AP-1) and NFkB and the start of the cascade of inflammation. AP-1 is another DNA caretaker or activator, similar to NFkB. Once again we can see the role of the NFkB family and its ability to start the inflammatory cascade.

STIMULATION OF
THE CHONDROCYTE VIA FREE RADICALS

Free radicals, those positively charged particles desperately looking to steal electrons from nearby molecules, may be produced by white blood cells fighting infections, mitochondrial energy production by-products, pollution, cigarette smoke, nitric oxide, or countless other irritants. Free radicals can directly damage joint collagen or sugar-proteins (glycoproteins) by ripping away their electrons and thereby inciting inflammation.

Through free radical-stimulated inflammation, cytokine molecules (TNF-alpha, IL-1 beta), and other enzymes (collageases) that directly impact collagen and extracellular matrix are produced and, in short, cause direct damage to the structures that keep joints healthy and working their best.

Inflammatory and anti-inflammatory messengers guide the joint toward pain or to peace and harmony. Now we have identified and are vigorously researching the NFkB family of DNA caretakers, or transcription factors, the central regulatory linchpin that controls the production of inflammatory molecules like COX-2, and bad prostaglandins (Li 2005). NFkB is a family of molecules that float around in the cytoplasm in an inactive state. I consider Nfat, SOX, SAF-1, and NFkB as DNA caretakers important for joint health. For simplicity, I call all these DNA caretakers the NFkB family of DNA caretakers. When stimulated, they have the ability to enter the nucleus and kick-start the production of inflammatory cytokine messengers, like matrix metalloproteinases, tumor necrosis factor, and interleukin-1 beta, which cause joint pain and destruction. The NFkBs are structurally similar, and SAF-1 and SOX are like cousins in my mind. See my website at www.healthyjointsforlife.com for additional information on these fascinating transcription factors.

As this book has tried to show, the far-reaching effects of these regulatory linchpins go beyond the joints. Joint pain, heart disease, and cancer are all intimately related to the NFkB family of DNA caretakers.

THE NITTY-GRITTY ON NFkB

NFkB normally exists in an inactive state, floating around in the cytoplasm. It is composed of two subunits called Rel(A, B, or C) and p(50 or 52). Probably the most thoroughly investigated of the various subunit combinations is the RelA-p50 complex.

The RelA-p50 complex is active, unless it is inhibited or inactivated by the inhibitor kappa beta family of proteins (IkB). These proteins bind to the RelA-p50 and keep RelA p50 from going into the nucleus. Those of us with joint pain love our friend IkB's ability to stop NFkB, since this means inflammation is halted in its tracks. If our friend IkB keeps NFkB inactive, we have less joint pain.

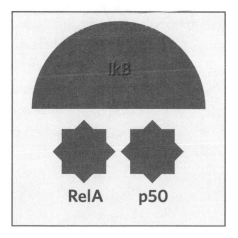

In order to activate RelA-p50, otherwise known as NFkB, our friend IkB must be physically removed from its attachment to the RelA-p50 complex. The archenemy of our friend IkB is a molecule called inhibitor kappa kinase, IkK. We do not like IkK, because it has the ability to remove our friend IkB from its attachment to RelA-p50. For those of you who are Superman fans, IkK is like kryptonite to our friend IkB. It weakens and incapacitates it. With our friend IkB removed from the previously inactive RelA-p50 complex, the invigorated and active RelA-p50 molecule is able to enter the nucleus, where it can activate DNA. This is extremely important to know for at least two reasons. If we can strengthen or increase the numbers of our friend IkB, we can subdue NFkB. If we can weaken or decrease the numbers of our archenemy IkK, then we can also help subdue NFkB. Do you see why it is so important that we know such intricate details about NFkB?

The magical way that our archenemy IkK works is by adding a phosphate group to our friend the IkB molecule, which is then a sitting duck for a process called ubiquitination. During the process of ubiquitination, a bunch of molecules of ubiquitin, a specific protein, are attached to the IkB-phosphate molecule, making it stick out like a sore thumb. This large complex, called a proteasome complex, is easily identified and degraded into small proteins by another enzyme. Our friend the IkB molecule is therefore degraded, and RelA-p50 is able to enter the nucleus, attach, and activate DNA. On the left of the diagram that follows, our friend IkB is inhibiting a RelA-p50 molecule. Our joints are happy. Moving left to right, our archenemy IkK then adds two Ps (phosphates) to our friend IkB, causing it to fall off RelA-p50. On the right, the freed RelA-p50 can then enter the nucleus, where it can stimulate the DNA to start the inflammatory cascade. Our joints aren't nearly as happy.

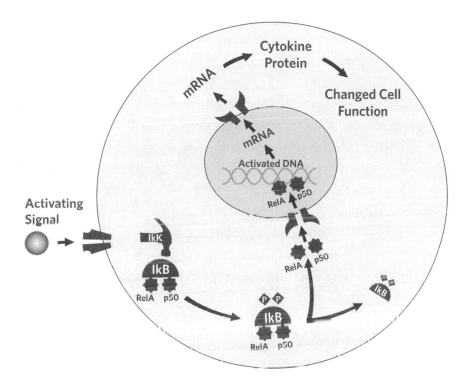

The NFkB molecule, in the form of RelA-p50, is able to enter the nucleus because a specific area of the NFkB protein sequence is exposed exactly where our friend the IkB molecule was detached. The NFkB protein sequence that is exposed, called the nuclear localization signal, is the appropriate key to unlock a nuclear pore, which then shuttles the NFkB molecule into the nucleus. Until our friend IkB is knocked off RelA-p50, the key to the nucleus is not exposed, so it can't unlock the nucleus membrane door, which is scientifically known as a nuclear pore.

Inside the nucleus other sequences of amino acids on the RelA-p50 molecule are able to identify the DNA genes that code for inflammatory molecules, like tumor-necrosis-factor-alpha (TNF-alpha), interleukins (IL), interferons (IFN), and the COX-2 and LOX enzymes. Through a yet to be discovered mechanism, NFkB unwinds the DNA, and the process for the production of inflammatory molecules begins. In an earlier chapter we learned about the important COX-2 enzyme. The COX-2 enzyme is a rather large complex protein that acts on arachidonic acid to produce "bad" prostaglandins, that is, those prostaglandins that induce inflammation. Incredibly enough, one of the large, complex proteins that NFkB controls is the COX-2 enzyme. If one could stop or slow down NFkB, then one would easily be able to decrease the amount of COX-2 enzyme available to cause inflammation through the pathways we initially learned about in Chapter 3 and were reacquainted with a few pages ago. That gives us two strategies to decrease "bad" prostaglandin production:

1. **Decrease the amount of omega-6 fatty acids** in the cell membranes, as omega-6s can act as building blocks for the pathway (omega-6 → arachidonic acid → "bad" prostaglandins).

2. **Stop NFkB from producing the COX-2 enzyme** that catalyzes the steps between arachidonic acid and "bad" prostaglandins. Now add TNF-alpha and IL-1 beta (other sinister inflammatory messengers) to the COX-2 enzyme and you are starting to understand the magnitude of the inflammatory response that NFkB can mount. Slow down the NFkB train and you have largely halted the excessive inflammatory process that leads to joint pain.

I've just explained to you how NFkB works to cause inflammation. Incredible stuff, wouldn't you say? But we can't stop there, because NFkB is also responsible for producing proteins that control the cell life cycle.

The inflammation hypothesis of aging states that cells, and by extension the human body, age as the inflammatory cycle gets out of balance (Chung 2001). Over time the inflammatory cycle gets more active, leading to cell-membrane, organelle, and DNA damage and an interruption of the normal cell cycle. The cell cycle is intrinsically coded in each cell's DNA. A cascade of events called apoptosis directs the cell to, in essence, commit suicide when its preprogrammed time is up. Cells need to die before their DNA mutates or turns cancerous. The process of apoptosis by itself is fascinating, working through a cascade of enzymes called caspases. If the caspase cascade is blocked, and the DNA is mutated, then the cell becomes immortal and grows out of control, causing cancer. NFkB is one of the prime agents directing the blocking of the caspase cascade. Our job is to influence NFkB so more of it stays inactive.

The sequence of reactions involved in the activation of NFkB is much more complicated than the basics I've just presented. For instance, there are other kinases besides our archenemy IkK that activate NFkB. MAP kinase (MAPK) is like a sinister brother to arch-enemy IkK. Adding another layer of complexity, some healthy and friendly protein messengers protect our friend IkB by inactivating archenemy IkK, therefore maintaining NFkB in its inactive state with our friend IkB attached.

RelA has two brothers, B and C, and p50 has a sister, p52. I hate to tell you, but p50 has some cousins, too! I'm not going to introduce you to all of them. RelB-p52 is another NFkB variant that is acti-vated by a relative of archenemy IkK, NFkB inducing kinase (NIK). Unfortunately, the dastardly IkK has several other cousins, as well. And that doesn't bring into play SOX and Nfat!

I've said many times before that the body is amazing and complex. You and I don't have to know all the minute details, but we cer-tainly can get a general feeling for the concepts. I will leave it at this: Control NFkB and we control the inflammatory process. Control that process and we quell joint pain. All the tactics I've presented in the *Healthy Joints for Life* program work toward affecting inflammatory pathways, messengers, and especially the NFkB family.

THE SCIENCE BEHIND SUPPLEMENTS

LUTEIN AND ASTAXANTHIN

Research has show that both lutein and astaxanthin possess powerful effects against NFkB. They work by decreasing transcellular H_2O_2. H_2O_2 has the extraordinary ability to stimulate NFkB, which leads to inflammation. Restricting H_2O_2 levels is a powerful tool for suppressing NFkB. When NFkB is suppressed, so are the inflammatory cytokines, like TNF-alpha, COX-2, IL-1 beta, that NFkB regulates. Lutein and astaxanthin are joint healthy.

VITAMIN B$_6$

In 2005 Japanese scientists established that vitamin B_6 is able to suppress NFkB activation in macrophages (a type of white blood cell that migrates to the joint as part of the inflammatory cascade).

VITAMIN D

I am particularly interested in vitamin D because it has such a pivotal role in calcium metabolism (and therefore bone health), as well as white blood cell immune function (and therefore possible joint inflammation). Moreover, we are learning that vitamin D fulfills an extremely important role in general immune function, mood control, muscle strength, athletic performance, insulin regulation, blood pressure control, heart health, and cancer protection. Vitamin D can regulate one thousand genes!

The fact that physicians are seeing an epidemic of vitamin D deficiency is alarming. One of the problems is that no one knows the optimal blood level of vitamin D. After deliberating on the medical literature and weighing clinical experience, the Vitamin D Council is recommending blood levels of 50 ng/ml (25-hydroxy vitamin D), which is probably much higher than your medical doctor will recommend at your annual physical. Professor Robert Heaney of Creighton University has determined that 5000 IU of vitamin D_3 are necessary to maintain a level of 50 ng/ml. Taking an inexpensive (not cheap just inexpensive since vitamin D_3 isn't costly) supplement of vitamin D_3 or getting sufficient sunlight makes it easy to obtain an appropriate blood level of vitamin D. How do you judge sufficient sunlight exposure? Ten to fifteen minutes of sunlight for a fair-skinned individual will create nearly 10,000 IU of vitamin D_3. The USDA presently recommends 400 IU of vitamin D_3 per day, and laboratories routinely assign a "normal" value of 35 ng/ml! State-of-the-art recommendations are therefore vastly different, and I have no doubt that USDA recommendations will change in the future.

As an example of the epidemic nature of vitamin D deficiency, the NHANES III (National Health and Nutrition Examination Survey) showed that in the United States, 60 percent of women and 50 percent of men have levels below 30 ng/ml. This obviously means that vitamin D deficiency is at epidemic proportions.

The body can make its own vitamin D through exposure to ultraviolet light B (UVB) in sunlight. In the deep basal level of skin, through UVB stimulus a cholesterol derivative called 7-dehydrocholesterol is converted into vitamin D_3 (cholecalciferol). The amount of sunlight necessary for sufficient production of D_3 depends on skin pigmentation, as well as the type of sun exposure. Darker-skinned people need longer sun exposure. Seasons, latitude, and altitude all influence the "potency" of the sun. In winter, for example, the sun isn't as strong. The sun is stronger in areas located around the equator, as well as at higher altitudes. Although the "Mile High City" of Denver, Colorado, and Richmond, Virginia, are at approximately the same latitude, Denver's altitude means that the sun's effects are stronger there.

Dr. Cannell, author of *Athlete's Edge: Faster, Quicker, Stronger with Vitamin D,* reports that, in general, if your shadow is longer than you are, then the sun is not potent enough to produce vitamin D_3.

Vitamin D can also be obtained through diet. However, trying to get vitamin D through diet is difficult, because few foods contain significant amounts. A teaspoon of cod liver oil boasts over 1000 IU, while fatty fish, like salmon, tuna, and mackerel, have significantly smaller amounts. Beef liver, eggs, and cheese contain even smaller amounts. None of these foods, unless consumed daily and in quantity, can provide sufficient amounts of vitamin D_3 to achieve my recommended doses.

If someone is completely without sunlight, then vitamin D_3 needs to be ingested in order for the active form of vitamin D to be synthesized. This is not difficult, because supplements of D_3 are readily available and are inexpensive.

Changes to vitamin D occur in the skin first (as described above), the liver second, and finally in the kidneys. After forming in the skin, vitamin D_3 is hydroxylated (an OH group is added) in the liver to form 25-hydroxy vitamin D (this is the type of vitamin D measured in a blood test), and then it is hydroxylated again in the kidney to form 1,25-dihydroxy vitamin D, or *active* vitamin D (calcitriol). Most physicians don't realize that vitamin D metabolism occurs in other tissues besides the skin, the liver, and the kidneys, such as the breasts, the prostate, the muscles, the heart, and white blood cells (specifically macrophages). This is why vitamin D is so important to so many system functions.

Active vitamin D is particularly important for bone health and muscular contraction because of its effects on calcium levels. Active vitamin D keeps parathyroid hormone from removing calcium from bone and helps the intestines absorb calcium. The hardness of bone is intimately related to the molecular storage of calcium as hydroxyapatite. Without calcium, bones weaken and osteoporosis develops.

Calcium ion flow into muscle cells is responsible for the electrical activation of muscular contraction. Too much calcium flow into muscle cells and tetany, or spasm, occurs, while too little calcium flow and no muscular contraction occurs.

Active vitamin D functions by binding to a specific receptor, called, aptly enough, the vitamin D receptor. These vitamin D receptors are located in the nucleus of many cell types, including intestine, bone, kidney, and parathyroid, where calcium can be stringently regulated. Too much calcium in your bloodstream is extremely dangerous, because fatal heart arrhythmias can occur. The bones contain the body's largest deposit of calcium, so bone strength and musculoskeletal health are dependent on sufficient levels of vitamin D. Joints cannot be healthy without vitamin D. In children, a lack of vitamin D leads to rickets, which is typically characterized by bowed legs.

White blood cells are also influenced by vitamin D. As we learned earlier, white blood cells called macrophages are potent inflammatory cells. When summoned by the inflammatory cytokines, they can migrate to joints and cause inflammation. Vitamin D's inhibitory effect on NFkB in macrophages is, therefore, another one of its important functions.

If you are fair skinned, make sure to get ten to fifteen minutes of sunlight daily. You will need more sun exposure if you are darker skinned. If that's not possible, then you should take about 5000 IU of vitamin D daily, according to the Vitamin D Council. (See Dr. Cannell's 2011 book, *Athlete's Edge: Faster, Quicker, Stronger with Vitamin D*, noted in the resources, for a discussion of skin cancer, vitamin D, and sun exposure.) Supplementing at higher dosages, unless doctor recommended for documented low blood levels of vitamin D, is not recommended. Toxicity does not occur easily with vitamin D, but that doesn't mean we should be careless. A baseline blood level of 25-hydroxy vitamin D should be obtained (not 1,25-dihydroxy vitamin D), and depending on your level, an appropriate amount of vitamin D_3 should be taken. That amount will probably be about 5000 IU, but it may vary related to your size. Vitamin D_3 should be taken daily unless you can get the equivalent amount of sun. Naturally, if the determined baseline level were high, you wouldn't supplement with vitamin D_3. It is highly unlikely this will be the case. Be mindful of summer and winter sunlight levels, as well as variation in sun exposure in different geographical areas.

John Cannell, M.D., states in his 2011 book, *Athlete's Edge: Faster, Quicker, Stronger with Vitamin D*, that vitamin D_3 is very safe. Deep sunburns generate only 50,000 IU of vitamin D, and it would take the ingestion of nearly sixteen bottles of 250-count 1000 IU capsules before toxicity would occur. Regardless of vitamin D_3's general safety, care is always prudent, because vitamin D toxicity leads to high calcium levels, heart arrhythmias, as well as nausea, vomiting, and kidney failure.

Recently, I've seen a high proportion of female patients with low vitamin D levels, below 10 ng/ml. It is not unusual for doctors to place these vitamin D–deficient patients on 50,000 IU three times per week until their blood tests reflect sufficient levels. Dosing continues until normal blood levels of vitamin D are documented. Some of my patients have been very skeptical of taking vitamin D_3 supplements, so let me share this study with those who may question the overall significance of this vitamin.

A joint study (Richards 2007) by researchers from the United States and Britain and involving 2,160 women showed that vitamin D levels correlated with longevity. This study established that the ends of chromosomes, which are called telomeres, shorten with each cell replication and thus are indicators of age. The study found that women with the lowest vitamin D levels had telomeres that resembled those of women five years older.

Remember, too, that vitamin D works in cells to help prevent cancer, improves immune function against infections, such as the flu, and appears to improve athletes' performance. Have I convinced you to take vitamin D yet?

VITAMIN E

Although alpha-tocopherol has been shown in studies to inhibit the inflammatory messengers lipoxygenase, phospholipase, MMP-19, and collagenase, it is the gamma-tocotrienol subclass that has garnered more recent attention. Researchers from opposite sides of the world published results in the years 2007 to 2009 documenting vitamin E, subclass tocotrienol, as a dominant NFkB suppressor. Of all the tocotrienols, gamma-tocotrienol is the most potent NFkB blocker. Researchers in Taiwan found that the tocotrienol-rich part of palm oil possessed potent anti-inflammatory activity via the suppression of NFkB, iNO3, and COX-2. At the University of Texas, researchers went so far as to show that gamma-tocotrienols abolished NFkB activation, while tocopherols (the other vitamin E subclass) did not.

I'm excited by this research, which revealed gamma-tocotrienol as a significant anti-inflammatory and inhibitor of NFkB. As an added benefit, gamma-tocotrienols also inhibit HMG-CoA reductase, the key rate-limiting enzyme of cholesterol synthesis. Making cholesterol takes a number of steps/sequential reactions. The rate-limiting enzyme is the key step in controlling how fast the reaction occurs. For those with cholesterol problems, gamma-tocotrienol may be a reasonable part of your cholesterol management program. Vitamin E supplementation above 400 IU has been associated with heart disease so my recommendations are significantly less.

GRAPE SEED EXTRACT

The proanthocyanidins (PACs) of grape seed extract are responsible for significant benefits. PACs have the ability to modulate the production of advanced glycation end products (AGEs). As you recall, glycation is the process of abnormal bonding of sugar to substances, with the unfortunate result that they become sticky, stiff, and inflexible. This can be extremely damaging to structures susceptible to AGEs, like blood vessel walls (Li 2011). Tissues containing collagen, such as skin, tendons, cartilage, vessel walls, and muscle, would also be potential places for deleterious glycation. Because PACs have the ability to help prevent glycation, they are considered joint healthy for tendons, cartilage, and muscle. The cause of osteoarthritis is related in part to cartilage collagen glycation, which stiffens the cartilage, decreasing its mechanical ability to tolerate stress. Meanwhile, glycation of ligaments reduces flexibility and adds to stiffness. Preventing glycation is, therefore, quite important if you are fighting joint pain. The heroic ability of PACs to stop the formation of AGEs is exactly why PACs are so important to cardiovascular health. A sticky, stiff, glycated vessel wall is sure to clog. PACs also have the ability to block NFkB and, therefore, the expression of iNOS and COX-2, especially in skin, which will prevent wrinkles.

It has been determined that PACs are great antioxidants. Antioxidants work by providing electrons to destructive substances called free radicals, which would otherwise steal electrons from healthy molecules, thereby damaging them. We need to be particularly concerned about the fact that free radicals can damage DNA and cell membranes. This process can lead to inflammation and other worrisome processes, like cancer.

RESVERATROL

GlaxoSmithKline bought Sirtris Pharmaceutical in 2008 based largely on the molecule resveratrol. Sirtris founder, Dr. David Sinclair, is a leading investigator of a protein enzyme called Silent Information Regulator Two (SIRT1), which resveratrol can activate (Milne 2007).

Early research has indicated that resveratrol, via its effect on SIRT1, fights against inflammation and facilitates metabolism. Sirtuin (SIRT) is the family of enzymes that catalyze gene splicing, control apoptosis, and effect energy metabolism. These enzymes are thought to be important for extending life. Sirtuin is shortened to SIRT, and there is more than one enzyme in the family, hence the number following the name. Resveratrol's association with NFkB and SIRT puts it in the same company as two of the most exciting players in molecular biology.

Some of the excitement concerning resveratrol relates to its use as a potential treatment for diabetes and cancer. Even more eye-opening and tantalizing are the reports on resveratrol as a possible life extender, because of its lengthening effects on the life span of yeast (Sinclair 2003), fruit flies (2004), fish (2006), and honey bees (2012). In 2006 Sinclair also discovered positive effects in rats that were supplemented with resveratrol.

You should know that along with the extraordinary claims surrounding resveratrol, there are also many scientific doubters. Recently, concerns have surfaced about resveratrol's ability to trigger a response from SIRT (which in turn suppresses NFkB), and it has been argued that Sinclair's original experiments were marred by defects in the fluorophores, fluorescent markers central to the experimental design. Recent discoveries of the falsification of data on this same subject (in a lab completely separate from Sinclair's) by a University of Connecticut researcher, Dr. Dipak Das, have led to further skepticism. I'll spare you the gory chemical details, just this one time. Suffice it to say that it is important for all of scientific research to be corroborated by independent examination, so I am sure we have not heard the last concerning research on resveratrol. Despite the concerns of some, and the deceit of others, there remains a large amount of research demonstrating that resveratrol and grape seed extract block NFkB. Therefore, they remain prime candidates for fighting inflammation. Liu (2010) showed resveratrol specifically protected cartilage by neutralizing

AGEs and blocking NFkB. Enough independent labs have done favorable research to have me optimistic, with a bit of healthy skepticism!

CURCUMIN

Various modifications have been made to curcumin in an attempt to make it more potent. Dimethoxy curcumin, a synthetic curcumin analog with higher metabolic stability, was shown by Pae in a 2008 Korean study to inhibit nitric oxide and NFkB more effectively than curcumin alone. Another analog, called EF24, is ten times as potent as curcumin.

A DYNAMIC DUO: RESVERATROL AND CURCUMIN

Cells in the synovium produce cytokines, notably TNF-alpha and IL-1 beta. These sinister cytokines stimulate cartilage cells to produce matrix metalloproteinases (MMPs) and COX-2, which give rise to cartilage matrix degeneration, joint inflammation, and joint destruction. Cartilage cell death is even prompted by IL-1 beta.

It is now known that cartilage matrix components, like type II collagen, are regulated by the "master" cartilage DNA caretaker, transcription factor SOX-9. I know it isn't going to surprise you when I tell you that "grand master" NFkB also plays a significant role in influencing SOX-9.

In the commentary on resveratrol and curcumin in the above two sections, it is noted that these phytonutrients, independently, are cartilage protective via their effects on NFkB. A 2008 German study by Csaki reported that together resveratrol and curcumin have a synergistically protective effect on cartilage. I am not indicating an additive effect. I mean synergistic . . . exponential!

BOSWELLIA

I have been impressed with the anti-inflammatory action of boswellia. Early studies linked boswellia's anti-inflammatory effect to the inhibition of the 5-LOX enzyme, thereby limiting leukotriene production. It is also felt that the COX-2 enzyme is affected.

Siemoneit's study in *Biochemical Pharmacology* (2008) showed that AKBA, a boswellia derivative, inhibited COX-1 but affected COX-2 to a much lesser extent. Other studies in 2007 (Moussaieff) found that a boswellic acid derivative, called incensole, inhibited NFkB, while a 2006 study from Ohio State University (Roy) concluded that AKBA inhibits TNF-alpha and MMPs, which degrade cartilage matrix. These studies reveal that boswellia does not appear to act as an anti-inflammatory by directly blocking the COX-2 enzyme, but rather by blocking LOX, TNF-alpha, and NFkB. In choosing a boswellia supplement it is important to check for AKBA content.

POMEGRANATE

I am intrigued by the Case Western Reserve University study (Ahmed 2005) that showed that pomegranate fruit extract inhibited NFkB– and IL-1 beta–induced cartilage breakdown. It prevented NFkB from binding to chondrocytes' DNA, and therefore MMP-1, MMP-3, and MMP-13 were all down-regulated, meaning that proteoglycan (GAGs) matrix, the treelike scaffold of cartilage structure, was saved from MMP enzymatic breakdown. Pomegranate is a promising supplement for those with osteoarthritis.

GINGER

Altman and Marcussen published a randomized double-blind, placebo-controlled study in *Arthritis Rheumatology* in 2001. In this study of 261 patients with knee osteoarthritis, nearly two-thirds of the patients responded to ginger extract. A 2006 Australian study by Aktan, conducted on murine macrophages, showed that a gingerol metabolite, RAC-[6]-dihydroparadol, and a synthetic analog called Capsarol (capsaicin/gingerol) inhibited NFkB and that in turn iNOS production was reduced, so that nitric oxide production was also controlled.

Ahmed et al. in 2008 and 2000 found that animals fed ginger had less lipid peroxidation (unhealthy fat breakdown) and oxidative stress (the type of stress that activates NFkB). Ginger appears to be an effective antioxidant and anti-inflammatory, as well as selective NFkB inhibitor. And a Japanese study done in 2007 (Ishiguro) showed that [6]-gingerol inhibited gastric cancer cell NFkB activation. Because NFkB can prevent cell death, and gingerol can stop NFkB, it was found to have a damaging effect on gastric cancer cell viability.

GREEN TEA

In 2009 Rasheed from the University of South Carolina School of Medicine showed that EGCG in green tea inhibits advanced glycation end products (AGEs), as well as TNF-alpha and MMP-13 in human cartilage cells.

In Chapter 4 I mentioned the Akhtar (2011) and Katiyar (2011) studies that showed EGCG blocked NKkB and twenty-nine inflammatory proteins produced by NFkB. An English study from 2002 (Adcocks) concluded that the catechins in green tea inhibited the breakdown of type II collagen and proteoglycan—two very important matrix components of joint cartilage. Furthermore, a Japanese study in 2007 (Hou) found that prodelphinidin B-4 3'-O-gallate (PBG), another green tea gallate, similar to EGCG, blocked activation of NFkB and thereby down-regulated COX-2 and iNOS, the two enzymes of inflammation we've learned so much about in the last several chapters!

GLUCOSAMINE AND CHONDROITIN

In general, results from European studies on glucosamine and chondroitin are definitely more favorable than those from American studies. One landmark 2002 European study from the Czech Republic (Pavelka) evaluated 202 patients and found that taking glucosamine for three years retarded the progression of knee arthritis. This is truly earth-shattering news with incredible implications. If you can slow the progression of cartilage breakdown, you can save hundreds of thousands of patients from years of pain and perhaps surgery. Many doctors, including me, were and remain skeptical of the results of that study. I should also mention that the study showed that there was improvement in symptoms in 20 to 25 percent of patients, in addition to the structural benefits.

A Spanish study from 2007 that evaluated 318 patients concluded that 1500 mg of glucosamine sulfate was more effective than placebo in treating osteoarthritis symptoms. Spanish (Monfort) and Swiss (Uebelhart) studies from 2008 showed that chondroitin had slight to moderate efficacy in treating the symptoms of osteoarthritis. The Swiss study suggested that 800 mg was nearly as effective as 1200 mg and that alternating three months on and three months off was just as effective as continuous treatment.

The European research is thought to be so convincing that in Europe glucosamine and chondroitin (DONA) are prescription medications and are highly recommended for the treatment of osteoarthritis. Meanwhile, in the United States, the National Institutes of Health (NIH), in its 2008 study called the Glucosamine/chondroitin Arthritis Intervention Trial (GAIT), evaluated 1,583 patients and concluded that, overall, glucosamine and chondroitin did *not* reduce pain compared to placebo. Celebrex, a common anti-inflammatory available only by prescription, on the other hand, did. Specific numbers show that 60.1 percent of placebo-taking patients were helped, while 66.6 percent of glucosamine chondroitin–taking patients were helped, and 70.1 percent of patients on Celebrex were helped. Because of statistical analysis, the difference between placebo (60.1 percent) and glucosamine/chondroitin (66.6 percent) was not determined to be significant. The 10 percent difference between placebo and Celebrex was significant, however.

Sometimes statistics can be confusing. The bottom line is that the GAIT study concluded that, although the numbers were better for patients taking glucosamine and chondroitin, the percentage difference was not enough to say that it was more than simply chance that glucosamine and chondroitin reduced pain compared to placebo. The most interesting part of the study, however, pertained to the subset of patients with moderate to severe arthritis. Of the total 1,583 patients, 354 had moderate to severe arthritis. More of those patients responded favorably to glucosamine/chondroitin (79 percent) than did the patients who were treated with Celebrex. It would seem that patients with milder arthritis do not see as good results when treated with glucosamine and chondroitin as patients with moderate to severe arthritis. The follow-up study, done in 2010 by Sawitzke, to the above mentioned 2008 GAIT study enrolled 662 patients with moderate to severe knee osteoarthritis. The results were unimpressive for the "dependable use" of Celebrex, glucosamine alone, or glucosamine and chondroitin as a reliever of the symptoms of osteoarthritis.

Combining all the evidence, I have some reservations but come down favorably on the side of glucosamine and chondroitin. Personally, I find glucosamine and chondroitin helpful in my own treatment. I have also seen hundreds of patients express improvement. The European study in 2002 by Pavelka, showing a cessation in the progression of osteoarthritis, and the specific improvement in moderate to severe arthritis patients in the 2008/2010 NIH GAIT studies are a bit perplexing, but overall, I feel that glucosamine and chondroitin should be part of a joint-healthy supplement program. Another 2010 study from Belgium (Scholtissen), revealing that glucosamine sulfate is highly cost-effective over a six-month period (the length of the study), is the icing on the cake. You can consider taking a supplement with glucosamine and chondroitin in the same pill. The Swiss study that I alluded to earlier (Uebelhart 2008) indicated that it might be possible to take the supplement chondroitin for three months on and three months off and achieve the same results as taking the supplement continuously.

LICORICE

The ethanol-extracted roasted licorice reduced prostaglandin and nitric oxide production. It also inhibited NFkB by preventing our friend IkB, the molecule that inactivates NFkB, from being degraded. Isoliquiritigenin, a licorice component, worked wonders on cell adhesion molecules. Korean researchers (Kwon 2007) showed that isoliquiritigenin inhibited NFkB, which in turn prevented the DNA production of cell adhesion molecules. This is important for the inflammatory process of clogging or hardening of the arteries, known as atherosclerosis. In that process, white blood cells called macrophages are summoned to the arterial walls, where they can secrete cytokines. If the macrophages never adhere to the vessel walls, atherosclerosis, or the clogging of blood vessels, never occurs. This is a great example of how licorice can help prevent heart disease.

Real licorice can act like aldosterone, a hormone made in the adrenal gland that helps control the kidneys' filtering of sodium, potassium, and water. Aldosterone causes the absorption of sodium and the excretion (via urine) of potassium. Water follows the sodium and is reabsorbed into the circulation. Aldosterone, therefore, causes fluid retention and the wasting of potassium. If aldosterone levels get too high, potassium levels can be depleted and fluid retention can lead to high blood pressure. This explains my major concern with the side effect of licorice extracts.

SILYMARIN

University of Texas researchers (Manna 2000) have found that silymarin inhibits IkB and other molecules, like MAPK, that free NFkB to enter the nucleus. The long-known cytoprotective and anti-inflammatory effects of silymarin make it an attractive supplement for a joint-healthy lifestyle. Research that was conducted in India by Ashkavand in 2012 showed that silymarin was able to reduce inflammation-provoking IL-1 beta and the fibrillation of articular cartilage in rats with osteoarthritis. Silymarin has joint-specific anti-inflammatory value. Another 2012 study, this one by Malekinejad, found that silymarin works as a potent antioxidant, able to reverse some of the inflammatory molecular effects of diabetes.

GUGGULSTERONES

I am excited by the 2008 study (Lee) showing that gugguls inhibited NFkB– and IL-1 beta–induced MMPs in joint-lining synovial cells. They have also been shown to help maintain pancreatic beta cells and to retard diabetes, once again through the inhibition of NFkB (Lv 2008). One study found that cell type didn't matter. Gugguls stopped NFkB in leukemia cells and epithelial (tissue) cells, as well. The inflammatory stimulus, whether it is cigarette smoke, IL-1 beta, TNF-alpha, or various acids, wasn't a factor. Gugguls are versatile enough to stop NFkB no matter the cell type or stimulus (Shishodia 2003).

Gugguls stop inflammatory pathways in epithelial cells, cancer cells, synovial joint cells, as well as pancreatic cells and even bone cells. Incredibly, they also have the ability to keep white blood cells from differentiating into bone-resorbing cells, as seen in metastatic cancers, which is an indication that gugguls should be part of a cancer-free lifestyle (Ichikawa 2006).

BETAINE

Betaine is a really cool molecule because of the biochemical gymnastics it can do. If you're old enough to have seen Romanian gymnast Nadia Comaneci achieve a perfect ten at the 1976 Summer Olympics, then you'll understand what I mean when I say that betaine is like Nadia, because it can literally flip CH_3 groups perfectly to other molecules in the process of making, for instance, neurotransmitters, like dopamine and serotonin. Betaine also helps on the balance beam with the synthesis of glutathione and on the uneven bars with coenzyme Q10 synthesis, as well as with the synthesis of another supplement, melatonin. I also love that it can decrease heart-unhealthy homocysteine, lending a CH_3 group to make unhealthy homocysteine into healthy methionine. B_{12} and folate are the major enzymes for that pathway, but betaine is happy playing a secondary role, doing what it can for the team. Its role in maintaining glutathione levels helps with joint health. As you know, when glutathione levels wane, free radicals wreak havoc and stimulate NFkB activation. Betaine helps keep NFkB inactive, thereby down-regulating COX-2 and TNF-alpha. Joints love it when COX-2 and TNF-alpha are suppressed. So will you. This was all shown quite nicely in a 2007 Korean study by Go in *Biological & Pharmaceutical Bulletin*.

Betaine is a good antiaging molecule because of its effect on glutathione, free radicals, NFkB, and the resultant inflammatory molecules called cytokines. Methyl (CH_3) donors, like betaine, also protect DNA from mutating by way of a process called DNA methylation.

In that process, strong binding parts of DNA (Gs and Cs) are made weaker (like As and Ts). The weaker binding areas don't attract carcinogens and thereby prevent DNA from mutating.

KAVA

A 2009 Australian study (Sarris) of sixty patients taking water-extracted kava showed that kava did not cause liver damage. It was felt that the liver toxicity reported in 2001 was related to kava supplements that were extracted from the kava plant using alcohol or acetone and perhaps those derived from ground stems and leaves, which contain hepatotoxic pipermethystine. This liver toxicity was conspicuously geographic in nature, in that only westernized alcohol and acetone extraction techniques led to problems, while Pacific water extraction techniques were harmless, and thus it became known as the "Pacific kava paradox." In 2009 Teschke, who is perhaps the leading authority on this subject, showed that liver toxicity actually occurs with both the alcohol/acetone extraction techniques and the water extraction techniques. Teschke (2012) noted, "It appears that the primary cause of toxicity may reside in the time before the preparation of the various kava extracts, possibly attributed to poor quality of the raw material caused by mould hepatotoxins." I don't recommend Kava because of the toxicity concerns.

APPENDIX II

How the
Healthy Joints for Life Lifestyle Works To Battle Heart Disease and Decrease Cancer Risk

BY USING THIS GUIDE TO PREVENT JOINT PAIN, YOU WILL SEE TWO additional major health benefits. The *Healthy Joints for Life* lifestyle, which so effectively diminishes joint pain, also protects against heart disease and cancer. This should come as no surprise because we know that NFkB, the conductor of joint inflammation, also plays a key role in both heart disease and cancer.

Through the same mechanism of influencing NFkB, the *Healthy Joints for Life* lifestyle decreases the risk of heart disease and cancer. The trail of evidence in the scientific literature to substantiate the effects of this lifestyle on heart disease and cancer is considerable, and it continues to be exciting to anyone trying to remain on or move beyond the cutting edge when it comes to battling disease.

The *Healthy Joints for Life* lifestyle also fights obesity, which has been directly and indirectly linked to heart disease and cancer. The commentary on diet presented in this book probes the issue of controlling insulin levels; warns about the easily oxidized PUFAs; exposes the shortcomings of trans fats, processed meats, certain saturated fats, and omega-6/omega-3 imbalances; and delineates the steps that need to be taken to improve bad cholesterol levels (especially the oxidized LDL fraction).

BATTLING HEART DISEASE WITH THE *HEALTHY JOINTS FOR LIFE* DIET

Many view heart disease as an inflammatory disease of blood vessels. If the vessels that clog are the ones that deliver blood to the heart muscle itself, a part of the heart dies, and a cardiac infarction, or heart attack will occur. Chronic vascular inflammation orchestrated by NFkB is thought to be one cause of cardiovascular disease, or hardening of the arteries. Fighting this process is therefore incredibly important.

The *Healthy Joints for Life* diet recommends increasing omega-3 consumption while stabilizing omega-6s, eliminating trans fats, reducing oxidized PUFAs, and decreasing saturated fat consumption. It fits perfectly into a heart-healthy model. Controlling insulin by regulating carbohydrate consumption is an extremely valuable tool for lipid/cholesterol management, as well as for limiting blood vessel disease progression. Insulin stimulates the formation of HMG-CoA reductase, which is a critical enzyme in cholesterol synthesis. If HMG-CoA reductase levels increase, so will cholesterol levels including the most alarming subfraction, oxidized LDL. Insulin also has a direct effect on NFkB. An increase in NFkB levels in cells lining the blood vessels kick-starts the inflammatory process, leading to swelling and narrowing of the vessels. Insulin, therefore, plays an important role in how the blood vessel disease called atherosclerosis develops. Controlling insulin secretion via carbohydrate manipulation, one of the central tenets of the *Healthy Joints for Life* diet, therefore, is a straightforward strategy for helping to control heart disease.

Considerable information regarding cardiovascular health has been obtained from the Nurses' Health Study, which started in 1976 and has followed 121,700 female registered nurses in the years since. Nearly two hundred studies have been generated from this large cohort of patients. The results from subsequent follow-up studies performed decades after the initial study began showed that trans fat consumption increased heart disease and risk and polyunsaturated fat consumption (omega-3s and omega-6s) reduced heart disease and risks (Mozaffarian 2006). My dietary recommendations fit perfectly with this study's results, perhaps refining suggestions by recommending more omega-3s and fewer omega-6s.

A study of 40,230 male health professionals in the United States found that modest fish consumption (fish high in omega-3 polyunsaturated fats) was associated with a lower risk of heart disease (Virtanen 2008). It has become common knowledge that not all saturated fats have the same effect on LDL "bad" cholesterol. For example, stearic acid—a saturated fat with eighteen carbons, which is seen in higher concentration in grass-fed beef—has beneficial effects on LDL "bad" cholesterol. Meanwhile, shorter-length saturated fats of fourteen carbons (myristic) and sixteen carbons (palmitic) —both more commonly found in higher concentrations in grain-fed cows—do not have as favorable effects. Studies support my *Healthy Joints for Life* diet recommendations of avoiding grain-fed beef and substituting grass-fed beef when you choose beef (Daley 2010; Hunter 2010).

Stearic acid is also found in a food that is loved, or should I say worshipped, by many and is part of the *Healthy Joints for Life* diet recommendations—chocolate, specifically dark chocolate. In an article entitled "Chocolate and Prevention of Cardiovascular Disease: A Systematic Review," published in 2006 in *Nutrition & Metabolism,* Dr. Eric Ding tells you exactly why it is imperative for you to eat dark chocolate for heart health. You learned earlier in this book that cocoa is joint healthy. Once again joint health and heart health go hand in hand.

It turns out that cocoa has a substantial concentration of the beneficial saturated fat stearic acid, which is found in grass-fed cows and is heart-healthy. Cocoa also contains antioxidant PACs (proan-thocyanidins) and flavonols, including catechins, which have also achieved fame as the heart-healthy antioxidants found in green tea and red wine. These antioxidants stop platelet aggregation (clot-ting that leads to heart attacks) and inhibit inflammatory molecules called cytokines. Do I have to say any more to convince you to eat chocolate? Do it for your joints; do it for your heart!

Carbohydrates stimulate the inflammatory cycle and cholesterol production. Too much cholesterol, in particular, oxidized LDL "bad" cholesterol, can have a negative effect on your cardiovascular health. Too much sugar in your system can lead to AGEs, advanced glyca-tion end products, which in turn cause blood vessel walls to harden. Controlling insulin by regulating carbohydrate consumption controls AGEs, reduces LDL "bad" cholesterol, and protects blood vessels.

In 2010 Mozaffarian, of Harvard University, published a study analyzing all the randomized controlled trials on PUFAs as a replace-ment for saturated fats and concluded that indeed consuming PUFAs in place of saturated fats reduced coronary heart disease. The literature has shown that replacing a diet high in saturated fat with a high-carbohydrate diet is not nearly as good an option as replacing the saturated fats with polyunsaturated fats, namely omega-3s and omega-6s. The versatility of my joint-healthy diet shines brightly, in that it is not only joint-healthy but also heart-healthy. It is my opinion that by taking care of your joints, you will be helping your heart, as well. My suggestion of tilting the balance of PUFAs toward omega-3s and away from omega-6s will even fur-ther improve heart health.

REDUCING CANCER RISK WITH THE *HEALTHY JOINTS FOR LIFE* DIET

It is no mystery that unhealthy diets lead to obesity. Diet, obesity, and cancer are interrelated, directly and indirectly. An inappropriate diet leads to obesity, and that most certainly affects your chances of getting cancer. Diet leads to cancer via other mechanisms besides obesity, as well. Processed foods containing nitrites, like sausages and hot dogs, can cause cancer (Bingham 1996). Chemicals in red meat, which are broken down in our GI tract into known carcinogens, can cause cancer. The *Healthy Joints for Life* diet, which stresses fiber, fish, and white meats, along with a lower glycemic rainbow of fruits and vegetables, is the perfect diet to fight obesity and cancer.

The European Prospective Investigation into Cancer and Nutrition (EPIC) has shown how fiber (a joint-healthy diet recommendation) can reduce the risk of colon cancer. It also found that processed meats increased colon cancer risk even more than red meats. The joint-healthy diet I recommend doesn't include an abundance of either processed meat or red meat. Also, chicken does not appear to increase cancer risk, and fish appears to decrease risks (Norat 2005). We know that obesity in women leads to excessive estrogen levels, which in turn are associated with cancers, particularly breast cancer. The literature shows an increased risk of breast cancer with increased omega-6 fatty acid consumption and a decreased risk with increased omega-3 fatty acid consumption (Sonestedt 2008).

The *Healthy Joints for Life* diet helps manage weight, thereby decreasing the chances of developing obesity-related cancers. We stress balancing omega-6 and omega-3 fats. By emphasizing fiber, fish, white meat, fruits, and vegetables, while downplaying processed meats and red meats, we end up with addition by subtraction. Avoiding the "bad" cancer-causing foods and eating the nutrient-rich foods puts your body in a perfect position to avoid cancer.

BATTLING HEART DISEASE WITH THE *HEALTHY JOINTS FOR LIFE* EXERCISE PLAN

I don't think you will be surprised to learn that getting into shape is heart-healthy. In one study (Myers 2002) fitness was a better predictor of cardiac mortality than high blood pressure, cholesterol level, smoking, or diabetes. According to government estimates, nearly 70 percent of the adult population in the United States doesn't meet the minimum recommendations for exercise. The fact is that those who would benefit the most from exercise are those who go from never exercising to doing very light exercise. For this group, the risk for heart disease can decrease by as much as 45 percent with minimal effort. This concept of small change for big gain is especially important for joint pain patients to understand and embrace, because pain causes many who have joint problems to be sedentary. It's important to realize that even a program of mild exercise can yield major cardiovascular benefits. Ironically, those who go from moderate fitness to intense fitness show only mild improvement in reducing their risk of heart disease.

Your heart is a muscle, and it benefits from exercise, too. Muscles need to receive substantial amounts of oxygen and nourishment in order to work at their best. Exercise improves the ability of blood-delivering coronary arteries to dilate and deliver blood to the heart in particular (Duncker 2008). Exercise has specific molecular implications, and as usual, those involve DNA activation and protein synthesis. The end result is that exercise facilitates increased blood flow throughout the body.

In 2008 and 2009 Chinese investigators published a two-part update on exercise and cardiovascular disease in *Sports Medicine* that beautifully summarizes the molecular basis for the positive effects of exercise on heart disease (Leung 2008; Yung 2009). They highlighted the effects of exercise on the DNA of endothelial cells (the cells that line the blood vessel lumen). Exercise affected the genes that control cellular metabolism, inflammation, growth, and proliferation. Exercise improved metabolic efficiency, decreased inflammation by reducing TNF-alpha and IL-6, and fostered the formation of new blood vessels. The baseline blood pressure of heart blood vessels was lowered, thereby reducing the workload and the oxygen needs of the heart at rest and at work.

Clinical studies on exercise with women (Stampfer 2000 study of 84,129 women) and men (Myers 2002 study of 6,213 men) have determined that there are heart benefits for both genders. Studies showed that exercise decreases the risk of stroke, diabetes, hypertension, and coronary mortality. All that is needed is a little effort! You need to get motivated, get active. You know that doing modest exercise will reduce your joint pain. Just imagine, while reducing your joint pain, you'll also be doing great things for your heart. That is a fantastic bonus!

REDUCING CANCER RISK WITH THE *HEALTHY JOINTS FOR LIFE* EXERCISE PLAN

In polls about people's fears, cancer ranks among the most feared phenomena. Cancer is so prevalent that it has touched many families. Undoubtedly, the reality that chemo and radiation therapy are painful has reached nearly all Americans, either because a loved one has suffered or they have seen the highly publicized public interest stories. The financial burden of cancer is staggering; over $201 billion was spent on cancer care in 2008 alone (nhlbi.nih.gov/about/factpdf.htm). It is an understatement to describe cancer as a devastating medical disease that often has an equally devastating financial and emotional impact. Experts estimate that 25 percent of cancers are caused by obesity and living a sedentary lifestyle. Yet with a simple form of prevention dangling in front of our noses, we, as a country, still do not exercise.

In fact, the medical literature is teeming with studies documenting the ability of exercise to reduce the incidence of prostate, colon, breast, ovarian, cervical, and uterine cancers. Kenfield (2011), of Harvard, documented a 61 percent reduction in prostate cancer–specific death in men who exercised three hours per week, compared with men with prostate cancer who exercised less than one hour per week. Leslie Bernstein (1994), from USC, observed, "If one stands back and thinks about the biological mechanisms involved in breast cancer and takes what we know about physical activity, physical activity should reduce risk." Her research indicated a 50 percent reduction in breast cancer with four hours of exercise per week, a 30 percent reduction with three hours of exercise per week, and a reduced risk with only two hours of exercise per week. Overall, it does appear that the strongest positive effect for exercise in preventing breast cancer is among obese and postmenopausal women.

It is important to understand that cancer is a complex set of diseases with different etiologies involving different organs. Breast cancer is not the same as testicular cancer. Liver cancer differs from pancreatic cancer. And there can be multiple types of cancers in the same organ. But exercise can have a significant impact on many of these cancers, especially those related to obesity.

Another Harvard study, this one by Wyshak (2000), followed 5,400 female athletes and determined that there was a decrease in breast, cervical, ovarian, and uterine cancer rates in women who exercised compared to women of the same age who did not. It was shown that exercise decreased fat and estrogen levels, which have been strongly correlated with breast cancer.

Fifty-two studies from around the world investigating the link between exercise and colon cancer have been combined and analyzed and show a 24 percent reduced risk of colon cancer in those who exercise versus those who don't (Wolin 2009).

Exercise has been shown to lead to decreased NFkB, increased glutathione, and the increased production of DNA/cell repair enzymes. NFkB can stop apoptosis, so diminishing the effect of NFkB allows sufficiently damaged or mutated cells to die. Glutathione is our body's most powerful free radical scavenger, and it will buffer those free radicals produced abundantly in the mitochondria, which can damage cell membranes and DNA. Buffering free radicals stops the damage that leads to cancer-causing changes. Increasing the production of DNA/cell repair enzymes allows for the better supervision of mutations that occur and can be repaired.

As you exercise your painful joints in an attempt to reduce joint pain and improve the quality of your life, you may also be saving yourself from the devastation of cancer.

REDUCING CANCER RISK AND BATTLING HEART DISEASE WITH THE *HEALTHY JOINTS FOR LIFE* SUPPLEMENT RECOMMENDATIONS

The *Healthy Joints for Life* supplements are all subjects of impressive bench and/or clinical research, and they continue to be studied for their positive effects on health. While there certainly is a considerable difference between cancer prevention and cancer treatment, some of these supplements are under clinical trials as treatments for cancers. See the bibliography and www.healthyjointsforlife.com for a sampling of the many studies being done. Until all the studies are in, I am not saying that these supplements can cure cancer. And I am not saying that these supplements should take the place of any heart medication. But knowing how the disease processes work and what these supplements can do to fight inflammation, battle free radicals, reduce NFkB, promote normal cell life, protect the lining of vessels, reduce cholesterol, and so many other things suggests that these supplements should be a part of your arsenal, not only to combat joint pain but also to keep healthy for life.

If you are curious about the research, refer to the bibliography and go to www.healthyjointsforlife.com. Suffice it to say that there is a great deal of research happening—let this small sampling of scientific article titles demonstrate the incredible capabilities of supplements.

- "...Apoptosis in Human Lung Cancer Cells by Curcumin" (Saha 2010)
- "Green Tea...Implications for Cancer Prevention" (Wang 2010)
- "[Licorice] Inhibits Migration and Invasion of Prostate Cancer Cells..." (Kwon 2009)
- "Resveratrol: Biological and Pharmaceutical Properties as Anticancer Molecule" (Hsieh 2010)
- "[NAC] Blocks Formation of Cancer..." (Zahid 2010)
- "Cardiovascular Benefits of Garlic" (Brace 2002)

In an attempt to be concise, and to save you the time of wading through studies, take a look at the summary chart I've put together. A plus sign means a positive, or helpful, effect and a minus sign means no effect. Please don't interpret this chart as an indication that these supplements cure cancer or replace heart medication. They simply represent what I think of as an important piece of the puzzle in keeping you healthy.

SUPPLEMENT	EFFECT ON CANCER	EFFECT ON HEART DISEASE
Omega-3	+	+
Resveratrol	+	+
Curcumin	+	-
Ginger	+	+
Licorice	+	-/+
Pomegranate	+	+
NAC	+	+
Boswellia	+	+
Green tea	+	+
Mangosteen	+	+
Guggulsterones	+	+
Cocoa	+	+
Garlic	+	+
Ursolic acid	+	-

The joint-healthy supplements that I have recommended are impressive for their ability to fight joint pain. They become absolutely irresistible when you consider that they are heart-healthy and may help reduce cancer risk.

***

You are now armed with the program and the science behind it. If a little knowledge is a dangerous thing, then we're more than ready to combat joint pain.

I know you can do it—and remember, you're not in this alone. Stay in touch through www.healthyjointsforlife.com for additional information and helpful suggestions. We will celebrate our victories together.

The best of joint health to everyone.

RESOURCES

Books

Atkins, Robert C. *Dr. Atkins' New Diet Revolution*. Rev. ed. New York: HarperCollins, 2002.

Borushek, Allan, ed. *The Doctor's Pocket Calorie, Fat & Carbohydrate Counter*. Hudsonville, MI: Family Health Publications, 2002.

Bowden, Jonny. *Living the Low Carb Life*. New York: Sterling, 2004.

Cannell, John. *Athlete's Edge: Faster, Quicker, Stronger with Vitamin D*. San Dimas, CA: Here & Now Books, 2011.

Carpender, Dana. *500 Low-Carb Recipes*. Beverly, MA: Fair Winds Press, 2002.

Champe, P. C., and R. A. Harvey. *Lippincott's Illustrated Reviews: Biochemistry*. 2nd ed. Philadelphia: J.B. Lippincott, 1994.

Eades, Michael R., and Mary Dan Eades. *The Protein Power Lifeplan*. New York: Warner Books, 2000.

Heller, Rachael F., and Richard F. Heller. *The Carbohydrate Addict's Fat Counter*. New York: Signet, 2000.

———. *The Carbohydrate Addict's Gram Counter*. New York: Signet, 1993.

Roskoski, Robert, Jr., and Jack D. Herbert. *Biochemistry Review*. Philadelphia: Saunders, 1996.

Thompson, Rob. *The Glycemic-Load Diet*. New York: McGraw-Hill, 2006.

Websites

CommonSenseHealth.com

DietaryFiberFood.com

GenerationUcan.com

OmegaXL.com

WeightLossForAll.com

www.nal.usda.gov/fnic/foodcomp/Data/

BIBLIOGRAPHY

Several hundred references were used in formulating this book. In an attempt to keep the book manageable, yet thorough, the gold standard references (as well as those directly mentioned in the book) are included in this abbreviated bibliography. Please go to www.healthyjointsforlife.com for the complete compilation of references.

CHAPTER 1

Inflammation: The Cornerstone of Disease

Checker R. "Potent anti-inflammatory activity of ursolic acid, a triterpenoid antioxidant, is mediated through suppression of NF-kB, AP-1 and NF-AT," *PLoS One.* 7.2(2012):e31318.

Hogan PG. "Transcriptional regulation by calcium, calcineurin, and NFAT," *Genes Dev.* 17(2003):2205–32.

Kumar D. "Transcriptional synergy mediated by SAF-1 and AP-1: critical role of N-terminal polyalanine and two zinc finger domains of SAF-1," *J Biol Chem.* 284(3):1853–62.

Li Q, Withoff S, Verma IM. "Inflammation-associated cancer: NF-kappaB is the lynchpin," *Trends Immunol.* 2005 Jun;26(6):318–25.

Rao A. "Transcription factors of the NFAT family: regulation and function," *Annu Rev Immunol.* 15(1997):707–47.

Ray A. "An inflammation-responsive transcription factor in the pathophysiology of osteoarthritis," *Biorheology.* 45.3-4(2008):399–409.

Ridker, PM, Cook NR, Lee IM, Gordon D, Gaziano JM, Manson JE, Hennekens CH, Buring JE. "A randomized trial of low-dose aspirin in the primary prevention of cardiovascular disease in women," *N Engl J Med.* 2005 Mar 31;352(13):1293–304. Epub 2005 Mar 7.

Rodova M. "Nfat1 regulates adult articular chondrocyte function through its age-dependent expression mediated by epigenetic histone methylation," *J Bone Miner Res.* 26.8(2011): 1974–86.

Schroeppel JP. "Molecular regulation of articular chondrocyte function and its significance in osteoarthritis," *Histol Histopathol.* 26.3(2011):377–94.

Wang J, Gardner BM, Lu Q, Rodova M, Woodbury BG, Yost JG, Roby KF, Pinson DM, Tawfik O, Anderson HC. "Transcription factor Nfat1 deficiency causes osteoarthritis through dysfunction of adult articular chondrocytes," *J Pathol.* 2009 Oct;219(2):163–72.

Yudoh K, Trieu N, Nakamura H, Hongo-Masuko K, Kato T, Nishioka K. "Potential involvement of oxidative stress in cartilage senescence and development of osteoarthritis: oxidative stress induces chondrocyte telomere instability and downregulation of chondrocyte function," *Arthritis Res Ther.* 2005;7:R380–R391.

CHAPTER 2

Joints: How They Work and What Can Go Wrong

Fulcher GR, Hukins DWL, Shepherd DET. "Viscoelastic properties of bovine articular cartilage attached to subchondral bone at high frequencies," *BMC Musculoskeleta Disord.* 2009;10:61.

CHAPTER 3

Eat: Foods That Reduce Joint Pain

Checker R. "Potent anti-inflammatory activity of ursolic acid, a triterpenoid antioxidant, is mediated through suppression of NF-kB, AP-1 and NF-AT," *PLos One.* 7.2(2012):e31318.

Daley CA, Abbott A, Doyle PS, Nader GA, Larson S. "A review of fatty acid profiles and antioxidant content in grass-fed and grain-fed beef," *Nutr Journ.* 2010;9:10.

Devi Sampath P, Vijayaraghavan K. "Cardioprotective effect of alpha-mangostin, a xanthone derivative from mangosteen on tissue defense system against isoproterenol-induced myocardial infarction in rats," *J Biochem Mol Toxicol.* 2007;21(6):336-39.

Hasan N, Siddiqui MU, Toossi Z, Khan S, Iqbal J, Islam N. "Allicin-induced suppression of Mycobacterium tuberculosis 85B mRNA in human monocytes," *Biochem Biophys Res Commun.* 2007 Apr 6;355(2):471–76.

Hooper L, Kroon PA, Rimm EB, Cohn JS, Harvey I, Le Cornu KA, Ryder JJ, Hall WL, Cassidy A. "Flavonoids, flavonoid-rich foods, and cardiovascular risk: a meta-analysis of randomized controlled trials," *Am J Clin Nutr.* 2008 Jul;88(1):38–50.

Hung SH, Shen KH, Wu CH, Liu CL, Shih YW. "Alpha-mangostin suppresses PC-3 human prostate carcinoma cell metastasis by inhibiting matrix metalloproteinase-2/9 and urokinase-plasminogen expression through the JNK signaling pathway," *J Agric Food Chem.* 2009 Feb 25;54(4):1291–98.

Inzucchi SE, Sherwin RS. "Type 1 diabetes mellitus," in Goldman L, Schafer AI, eds. *Cecil Medicine.* 24th ed. Philadelphia, PA: Saunders Elsevier; 2011:chap 236.

Iwasaki Y, Kambayashi M, Asai M, Yoshida M, Nigawara T, Hashimoto K. "High glucose alone, as well as in combination with proinflammatory cytokines, stimulates nuclear factor kappa-B-mediated transcription in hepatocytes in vitro," *J Diabetes Complications.* 2007 Jan-Feb;21(1):56–62.

Kanner J. "Dietary advanced lipid oxidation endproducts are risk factors to human health," *Mol Nutr Food Res.* 2007 Sep;51(9):1094–101.

Lee J, Jung E, Kim Y, Lee J, Park J, Hong S, Hyun CG, Park D, Kim YS. "Rosmarinic acid as a downstream inhibitor of IKK-beta in TNF-alpha-induced upregulation of CCL11 and CCR3," *Br J Pharmacol*. 2006 Jun;148(3):366-75.

Lee KS. "Cocoa polyphenols inhibit phorbol ester-induced superoxidation formation in cultured HL-60 cells and expression of cyclooxygenase-2 and activation of NF-kappaB and MAPKs in mouse skin in vivo," *J Nutr*. 2006 May;136(5):1150-55.

Lee YR, Lee JH, Noh EM, Kim EK, Song MY, Jung WS, Park SJ, Kim JS, Park JW, Kwon KB, Park BH. "Guggulsterone blocks IL-1beta-mediated inflammatory responses by suppressing NF-kappaB activation in fibroblast-like synoviocytes," *Life Sci*. 2008 Jun 6;82(23-24):1203-9.

Murakami Y, Hirata A, Ito S, Shoji M, Tanaka S, Yasui T, Machino M, Fujisawa S. "Re-evaluation of cyclooxygenase-2-inhibiting activity of vanillin and guaiacol in macrophages stimulated with lipopolysaccharide," *Anticancer Res*. 2007 Mar-Apr;27(2):801-7.

Nakatani K, Yamakuni T, Kondo N, Arakawa T, Oosawa K, Shimura S, Inoue H, Ohizumi Y. "Gamma-Mangostin inhibits inhibitor-kappaB kinase activity and decreases lipopolysaccharide-induced cyclooxygenase-2 gene expression in C6 rat glioma cells," *Mol Pharmacol*. 2004 Sep;66(3):667-74.

Nakatani K. "Inhibition of cyclooxygenase and prostaglandin E2 synthesis by gamma-mangostin, a xanthone derivative in mangosteen, in C6 rat glioma cells," *Biochem Pharmacol*. 2002 Jan;63(1):73-79.

Nemoseck T, Cole S, Petrisko Y, Kern M. "Effects of agave nectar versus sucrose on weight gain, adiposity, blood glucose, insulin and lipid responses in mice," *FASEB J*. April 2010 24 (Meeting Abstract Supplement).

Okazaki M, Iwasaki Y, Jing H, Nishiyama M, Taguchi T, Tsugita M, Taniguchi Y, Kambayashi M, Hashimoto K. "Insulin enhancement of cytokine-induced coagulation/inflammation-related gene transcription in hepatocytes," *Endocr J*. 2008 Dec;55(6):967-75.

Oku T, Nakamura S. "Digestion, absorption fermentation and metabolism of functional sugar substitutes and their available energy," *Pure Appl. Chem*. Vol 74, No 7, pp 1253-1261, 2002.

Pathak, AK. "Ursolic acid inhibits STAT3 activation pathway leading to suppression of proliferation and chemo sensitization of human multiple myeloma cells," *Mol Cancer Res*. 2007 Sep;5(9):943-55.

Pergola C, Rossi A, Dugo P, Cuzzocrea S, Sautebin L. "Inhibition of nitric oxide biosynthesis by anthocyanin fraction of blackberry extract," *Nitric Oxide*. 2006 Aug;15(1):30-9.

Rimbach G, Melchin M, Moehring J, Wagner AE. "Polyphenols from cocoa and vascular health-a critical review," *Int J Mol Sci*. 2009 Nov 20;10(10):4290-309.

Shishodia S, Majumdar S, Banerjee S, Aggarwal BB. "Ursolic acid inhibits nuclear factor-kappaB activation induced by carcinogenic agents through suppression of IkappaBalpha kinase and p65 phosphorylation: correlation with down-regulation of cyclooxygenase 2, matrix metalloproteinase 9, and cyclin D1," *Cancer Res*. 2003 Aug 1;63(15):4375-83.

CHAPTER 4

Support: Supplements

Ahmed RS, Suke SG, Seth V, Chakraborti A, Tripathi AK, Banerjee BD. "Protective effects of dietary ginger (Zingiber officinales Rosc.) on lindane-induced oxidative stress in rats," *Phytother Res.* 2008 Jul;22(7):902–6.

Ahmed RS, Seth V, Banerjee BD. "Influence of dietary ginger (Zingiber officinales Rosc.) on antioxidant defense system in rat: comparison with ascorbic acid," *Indian J Exp Biol.* 2000 Jun;38(6):604–6.

Ahmed S, Wang N, Hafeez BB, Cheruvu VK, Haqqi TM. "Punica granatum L. extract inhibits IL-1 beta-induced expression of matrix metalloproteinases by inhibiting the activation of MAP kinases and NF-kappaB in human chondrocytes in vitro," *J Nutr.* 2005 Sep;135(9):2096–102.

Akhtar N. "Epigallocatechin-3-gallate suppresses the global interleukin-1-beta-induced inflammatory response in human chondrocytes," *Arthritis Res Ter.* 13.3(2011):R93. Print.

Aktan F, Henness S, Tran VH, Duke CC, Roufogalis BD, Ammit AJ. "Gingerol metabolite and a synthetic analogue Capsarol inhibit macrophage NF-kappaB-mediated iNOS gene expression and enzyme activity," *Planta Med.* 2006 Jun;72(8):727–34. Epub 2006 May 29.

Altman RD, Marcussen KC. "Effects of a ginger extract on knee pain in patients with osteoarthritis," *Arthritis Rheum.* 2001 Nov;44(11):2531–38.

Ashkavand Z, Malekinejad H, Amniattalab A, Rezaei-Golmisheh A, Vishwanath BS. "Silymarin potentiates the anti-inflammatory effects of Celecoxib on chemically induced osteoarthritis in rats," *Phytomedicine.* 2012 Aug 24.

Auvichayapat P, Prapochanung M, Tunkamnerdthai O, Sripanidkulchai BO, Auvichayapat N, Thinkhamrop B, Kunhasura S, Wongpratoom S, Sinawat S, Hongprapas P. "Effectiveness of green tea on weight reduction in obese Thais: A randomized, controlled trial," *Physiol Behav.* 2008 Feb 27;93(3):486–91.

Bailey RL, Dodd KW, Goldman JA, Gahche JJ, Dwyer JT, Moshfegh AJ, Sempos CT, Picciano MF. "Estimation of total usual calcium and vitamin D intakes in the United States," *J Nutr.* 2010 Apr;140(4):817–22. Epub 2010 Feb 24.

Borer KT. "Physical activity in the prevention and amelioration of osteoporosis in women: interaction of mechanical, hormonal and dietary factors," *Sports Med.* 2005;35(9):779–830.

Cao JJ, Nielsen FH. "Acid diet (high-meat protein) effects on calcium metabolism and bone health," *Curr Opin Clin Nutr Metab Care.* 2010 Nov;13(6):698–702.

Cardinali DP, García AP, Cano P, Esquifino AI. "Melatonin role in experimental arthritis," *Curr Drug Targets Immune Endocr Metabol Disord.* 2004 Mar;4(1):1–10.

Chen CH, Sheu MT, Chen TF, Wang YC, Hou WC, Liu DZ, Chung TC, Liang YC. "Suppression of endotoxin-induced proinflammatory responses by citrus pectin through blocking LPS signaling pathways," *Biochem Pharmacol.* 2006 Oct 16;72(8):1001–9.

Chopra A, Lavin P, Patwardhan B, Chitre D. "A 32-week randomized, placebo-controlled clinical evaluation of RA-11, an Ayurvedic drug, on osteoarthritis of the knees," *J Clin Rheumatol.* 2004 Oct;10(5):236–45.

Csaki C, Keshishzadeh N, Fischer K, Shakibaei M. "Regulation of inflammation signalling by resveratrol in human chondrocytes in vitro," *Biochem Pharmacol.* 2008;75:677–87.

Cutolo, M. "The melatonin-cytokine connection in rheumatoid arthritis," *ANN Rheum Dis.* 2005 August;64(8):1109–11.

Dulloo AG, Duret C, Rohrer D, Girardier L, Mensi N, Fathi M, Chantre P, Vandermander J. "Efficacy of a green tea extract rich in catechin polyphenols and caffeine in increasing 24-h energy expenditure and fat oxidation in humans," *Am J Clin Nutr.* 1999 Dec;70(6):1040–45.

Flynn A. "The role of dietary calcium in bone health," *Proc Nutr Soc.* 2003 Nov;62(4):851–58.

Garriguet D. "Bone health: osteoporosis, calcium and vitamin D," *Health Rep.* 2011 Sep;22(3):7–14.

Go EK, Jung KJ, Kim JM, Lim H, Lim HK, Yu BP, Chung HY. "Betiane modulates age-related NF-kappaB by thiol-enhancing action," *Biol Pharm Bull.* 2007 Dec;30(12):2244–49.

Harvey JA, Zobitz MM, Pak CY. "Dose dependency of calcium absorption: a comparison of calcium carbonate and calcium citrate," *J Bone Miner Res.* 1988 Jun;3(3):253–58.

Heaney RP, Dowell MS, Barger-Lux MJ. "Absorption of calcium as the carbonate and citrate salts, with some observations on method," *Osteoporos Int.* 1999;9(1):19–23.

Jerosch J. "Effects of Glucosamine and Chondroitin Sulfate on Cartilage Metabolism in OA: Outlook on Other Nutrient Partners Especially Omega-3 Fatty Acids," *Int J Rheumatol.* 2011;2011:969012. Epub 2011 Aug 2.

Kalpakcioglu B. "The role of melatonin in rheumatic diseases," *Infect Disord Drug Targets.* 2009 Aug;9(4):453–56.

Karch SB. *The Consumer's Guide to Herbal Medicine.* Hauppauge, NY: Advanced Research Press, 1999.

Katiyar SK. "Green tea: a new option for the prevention or control of osteoarthritis," *Arthritis Res Ther.* 13.4(2011):121. Print.

Kidd PM. "Bioavailability and activity of phytosome complexes from botanical polyphenols: the silymarin, curcumin, green tea, and grape seed extracts," *Altern Med Rev.* 2009 Sep;14(3):226–46.

Kimmatkar N, Thawani V, Hingorani L, Khiyani R. "Efficacy and tolerability of Boswellia serrata extract in treatment of osteoarthritis of knee–a randomized double blind placebo controlled trial," *Phytomedicine.* 2003 Jan;10(1):3–7.

Lee YR, Lee JH, Noh EM, Kim EK, Song MY, Jung WS, Park SJ, Kim JS, Park JW, Kwon KB, Park BH. "Guggulsterone blocks IL-1beta-mediated inflammatory responses by suppressing NF-kappaB activation in fibroblast-like synoviocytes," *Life Sci.* 2008 Jun 6;82(23–24):1203–9.

Li K, Kaaks R, Linseisen J, Rohrmann S. "Associations of dietary calcium intake and calcium supplementation with myocardial infarction and stroke risk and overall cardiovascular mortality in the Heidelberg cohort of the European Prospective Investigation into Cancer and Nutrition study (EPIC-Heidelberg)," *Heart.* 2012 Jun;98(12):920–25. doi: 10.1136/heartjnl-2011-301345.

Lv N. "Guggulsterone, a plant sterol, inhibits NF-kappaB activation and protects pancreatic beta cells from cytokine toxicity," *Mol Cell Endocrinol.* 2008 July 16;289(1–2):49–59.

Ma J, Johns RA, Stafford RS. "Americans are not meeting current calcium recommendations," *Am J Clin Nutr.* 2007 May;85(5):1361–66.

Majumdar AP, Banerjee S, Nautiyal J, Patel BB, Patel V, Du J, Yu Y, Elliott AA, Levi E, Sarkar FH. "Curcumin synergizes with resveratrol to inhibit colon cancer," *Nutr Cancer.* 2009;61(4):544–53.

Manna SK, Mukhopadhyay A, Aggarwal BB. "Resveratrol suppresses TNF-induced activation of nuclear transcription factors NF-kappa B, activator protein-1, and apoptosis: potential role of reactive oxygen intermediates and lipid peroxidation," *J Immunol.* 2000 Jun 15;164(12):6509–19.

Milne JC, Lambert PD, Schenk S, Carney DP, Smith JJ, Gagne DJ, Jin L, Boss O, Perni RB, Vu CB, Bernis JE, Xie R, Disch JS, Ng PY, Nunes JJ, Lynch AV, Yang H, Galonek H, Israelian K, Choy W, Iffland A, Lavu S, Medvedik O, Sinclair DA, Olefsky JM, Jirousek MR, Elliott PJ, Westphal CH. "Small molecule activators of SIRT1 as therapeutics for the treatment of type 2 diabetes," *Nature.* 2007 Nov 29;450(7170):712–16.

Muraki S, Yamamoto S, Ishibashi H, Oka H, Yoshimura N, Kawaguchi H, Nakamura K. "Diet and lifestyle associated with increased bone mineral density: cross-sectional study of Japanese elderly women at an osteoporosis outpatient clinic," *J Orthop Sci.* 2007 Jul;12(4):317–20.

Nagao T, Hase T, Tokimitsu I. "A green tea extract high in catechins reduces body fat and cardiovascular risks in humans," *Obesity (Silver Spring).* 2007 Jun;15(6):1473–83.

Poliquin S, Joseph L, Gray-Donald K. "Calcium and vitamin D intakes in an adult Canadian population," *Can J Diet Pract Res.* 2009 Spring;70(1):21–27.

Rasheed Z, Anbazhagan AN, Akhtar N, Ramamurthy S, Voss FR, Haqqi TM. "Green tea polyphenol epigallocatechin-3-gallate inhibits advanced glycation end product-induced expression of tumor necrosis factor-alpha and matrix metalloproteinase-13 in human chondrocytes," *Arthritis Res Ther.* 2009;11(3):R71.

Ridker PM, Cook NR, Lee IM, Gordon D, Gaziano JM, Manson JE, Hennekens CH, Buring JE. "A randomized trial of low-dose aspirin in the primary prevention of cardiovascular disease in women," *N Engl J Med.* 2005 Mar 31;352(13):1293–304. Epub 2005 Mar 7.

Rodríguez-Rodríguez E, Navia Lombán B, López-Sobaler AM, Ortega Anta RM. "Review and future perspectives on recommended calcium intake," *Nutr Hosp.* 2010 May-Jun;25(3):366–74.

Sawitzke AD, Shi H, Finco MF, Dunlop DD, Harris CL, Singer NG, Bradley JD, Silver D, Jackson CG, Lane NE, Oddis CV, Wolfe F, Lisse J, Furst DE, Bingham CO, Reda DJ, Moskowitz RW, Williams HJ, Clegg DO. "Clinical efficacy and safety of glucosamine, chondroitin sulphate, their combination, celecoxib or placebo taken to treat osteoarthritis of the knee: 2-year results from GAIT," *Ann Rheum Dis.* 2010 Aug;69(8):1459-64. doi: 10.1136/ard.2009.120469. Epub 2010 Jun 4.

Schreck R, Rieber P, Baeuerle PA. "Reactive oxygen intermediates as apparently widely used messengers in the activation of the NF-kappaB transcription factor and HIV-1," *EMBO J.* 1991 Aug;10(8):2247-58.

Shishodia S, Aggarwal BB. "Guggulsterone inhibits NF-kappaB and IkappaBalpha kinase activation, suppresses expression of anti-apoptotic gene products, and enhances apoptosis," *J Biol Chem.* 2004 Nov 5;279(45):47148-58.

Skenderi G. *Herbal Vade Mecum.* Rutherford, NJ: Herbacy Press, 2003.

Skidmore-Roth L. *Handbook of Herbs and Natural Supplements.* 2nd ed. St. Louis, MO: Mosby, 2003.

Sterk V, Büchele B, Simmet T. "Effect of food intake on the bioavailability of boswellic acids from a herbal preparation in healthy volunteers," *Planta Med.* 2004 Dec;70(12):1155-60.

Tripathi YB, Malhotra OP, Tripathi SN. "Thyroid Stimulating Action of Z-Guggulsterone Obtained from Commiphora mukul," *Planta Med.* 1984 Feb;50(1):78-80.

Uebelhart D. "Clinical review of chondroitin sulfate in osteoarthritis," *Osteoarthritis Cartilage.* 2008;16 Suppl 3:S19-21.

Vangsness CT Jr, Spiker W, Erickson J. "A review of evidence-based medicine for glucosamine and chondroitin sulfate use in knee osteoarthritis," *Arthroscopy.* 2009 Jan;25(1):86-94.

Yang JY, Della-Fera MA, Rayalam S, Ambati S, Hartzell DL, Park HJ, Baile CA. "Enhanced inhibition of adipogenesis and induction of apoptosis in 3T3-L1 adipocytes with combinations of resveratrol and quercetin," *Life Sci.* 2008 May 7;82(19-20):1032-39.

Yuan H, Ji WS, Wu KX, Jiao JX, Sun LH, Feng YT. "Anti-inflammatory effect of Diammonium Glycyrrhizinate in a rat model of ulcerative colitis," *World J Gastroenterol.* 2006 July 28;12(28):4578-81.

CHAPTER 5

Move: How Exercise Helps You Move Better and Feel Better

Burke J, Thayer R, Belcamino M. "Comparison of effects of two interval-training programmes on lactate and ventilatory thresholds," *Br J Sports Med.* 1994 Mar;28(1):18-21.

Carlsen H, Haugen F, Zadelaar S, Kleemann R, Kooistra T, Drevon CA, Blomhoff R. "Diet-induced obesity increases NF-kappaB signaling in reporter mice," *Genes Nutr.* 2009 Sep;4(3):215-22. Epub 2009 Aug 26.

Clement K, Langin D. "Regulation of inflammation-related genes in human adipose tissue," *J Intern Med.* 2007 Oct;262(4):422-30.

Kim W, Thambyah A, Broom N. "Does prior sustained compression make cartilage-on-bone more vulnerable to trauma?" *Clin Biomech (Bristol, Avon).* 2012 Aug;27(7):637-45. Epub 2012 Apr 24.

Salter RB. "The biologic concept of continuous passive motion of synovial joints. The first 18 years of basic research and its clinical application," *Clin Orthop Relat Res.* 1989 May;(242):12-25.

Smith LR, Trindade MC, Ikenoue T, Mohtai M, Das P, Carter DR, Goodman SB, Schurman DJ. "Effects of shear stress on articular chondrocyte metabolism," *Biorheology.* 2000;37(1-2):95-107.

Smith RL, Carter DR, Schurman DJ. "Pressure and shear differentially alter human articular chondrocyte metabolism: a review," *Clin Orthop Relat Res.* 2004 Oct;(427 Suppl):S89-S95.

Tremblay A, Simoneau JA, Bouchard C. "Impact of exercise intensity on body fatness and skeletal muscle metabolism," *Metabolism.* 1994 Jul;43(7):814-18.

Uzel SG, Buehler MJ. "Molecular structure, mechanical behavior and failure mechanism of the C-terminal cross-link domain in type I collagen," *J Mech Behav Biomed Mater.* 2011 Feb;4(2):153-61. Epub 2010 Jul 16.

APPENDIX I

The Cell Science Behind It All

Adcocks C, Collin P, Buttle DJ. "Catechins from green tea (Camellia sinensis) inhibit bovine and human cartilage proteoglycan and type II collagen degradation in vitro," *J Nutr.* 2002 Mar;132(3):341-46.

Ahmed RS, Suke SG, Seth V, Chakraborti A, Tripathi AK, Banerjee BD. "Protective effects of dietary ginger (Zingiber officinales Rosc.) on lindane-induced oxidative stress in rats," *Phytother Res.* 2008 Jul;22(7):902-6.

Ahmed RS, Seth V, Banerjee BD. "Influence of dietary ginger (Zingiber officinales Rosc.) on antioxidant defense system in rat: comparison with ascorbic acid," *Indian J Exp Biol.* 2000 Jun;38(6):604-6.

Ahmed S, Wang N, Hafeez BB, Cheruvu VK, Haqqi TM. "Punica granatrum L. extract inhibits IL-1beta-induced expression of matrix metalloproteinases by inhibiting the activation of MAP kinases and NF-kappaB in human chondrocytes in vitro," *J Nutr.* 2005 Sep;135(9):2096-102.

Akhtar N. "Epigallocatechin-3-gallate suppresses the global interleukin-1beta-induced inflammatory response in human chondrocytes," *Arthritis Res Ther.* 13.3(2011):R93. Print.

Aktan F, Henness S, Tran VH, Duke CC, Roufogalis BD, Ammit AJ. "Gingerol metabolite and a synthetic analogue Capsarol inhibit macrophage NF-kappaB-mediated iNOS gene expression and enzyme activity," *Planta Med.* 2006 Jun;72(8):727-34. Epub 2006 May 29.

Altman RD, Marcussen KC. "Effects of a ginger extract on knee pain in patients with osteoarthritis," *Arthritis Rheum.* 2001 Nov;44(11):2531–38.

Arterburn LM, Hall EB, Oken H. "Distribution, interconversion, and dose response of n-3 fatty acids in humans," *Am J Clin Nutr.* 2006 Jun;83(6 Suppl):1467S–1476S.

Ashkavand Z, Malekinejad H, Amniattalab A, Rezaei-Golmisheh A, Vishwanath BS. "Silymarin potentiates the anti-inflammatory effects of Celecoxib on chemically induced osteoarthritis in rats," *Phytomedicine.* 2012 Aug 24.

Bagga D, Wang L, Farias-Eisner R, Glaspy J, Reddy ST. "Differential effects of prostaglandin derived from omega-6 and omega-3 polyunsaturated fatty acids on COX-2 expression and IL-6 secretion," *PNAS.* 2003 Feb;100(4):1751–56.

Bianco FJ, Guitian R, Moreno J, de Toro FJ, Galdo F. "Effect of anti-inflammatory drugs on COX-1 and COX-2 activity in human articular chondrocytes," *J Rheumatol* 1999; 26:1366–73.

Cao J, Schwichtenberg KA, Hanson NQ, Tsai MY. "Incorporation and clearance of omega-3 fatty acids in erythrocyte membranes and plasma phospholipids," *Clin Chem.* 2006 Dec;52(12):2265–72. Epub 2006 Oct 19.

Champ PC, Harvey RA. *Lippincott's Illustrated Reviews: Biochemistry 2nd edition.* Lippincott Williams & Wilkins, 1994.

Chung HY, Kim HJ, Kim JW, Yu BP. "The inflammation hypothesis of aging: molecular modulation by calorie restriction," *Ann N Y Acad Sci.* 2001 Apr;928:327–35.

Clandinin MT, Foot M, Robson L. "Plasma membrane: can its structure and function be modulated by dietary fat?" *Comparative Biochemistry and Physiology Part B: Comparative Biochemistry.* 1983;76(2):335–39.

Csaki C, Keshishzadeh N, Fischer K, Shakibaei M. "Regulation of inflammation signalling by resveratrol in human chondrocytes in vitro," *Biochem Pharmacol.* 2008;75:677–87.

Csaki C., Mobasheri A, Shakibaei M. "Synergistic chondroprotective effects of curcumin and resveratrol in human articular chondrocytes: inhibition of IL-1beta-induced NF-kappaB-mediated inflammation and apoptosis," *Arthritis Res Ther.* 2009;11(6):R165.

Fan YY, Ly LH, Barhoumi R, McMurray DN, Chapkin RS. "Dietary docosahexaenoic acid suppresses T cell protein kinase C theta lipid raft recruitment and IL-2 production," *J Immunol.* 2004 Nov 15;173(10):6151–60.

Go EK, Jung KJ, Kim JM, Lim H, Lim HK, Yu BP, Chung HY. "Betiane modulates age-related NF-kappaB by thiol-enhancing action," *Biol Pharm Bull.* 2007 Dec;30(12):2244–49.

Goldring MB, Berenbaum F. "The regulation of chondrocyte function by proinflammatory mediators: prostaglandins and nitric oxide," *Clin Orthop Relat Res.* 2004 Number 427S, pp. S37–S46.

Hou DX, Luo D, Tanigawa S, Hashimoto F, Uto T, Masuzaki S, Fujii M, Sakata Y. "Prodelphinidin B-4 3'-O-gallate, a tea polyphenol, is involved in the inhibition of COX-2 and iNOS via the downregulation of TAK1-NF-kappaB pathway," *Biochem Pharmacol.* 2007 Sep 1;74(5):742–51. Epub 2007 Jun 14.

Hwang DH, Chanmugam PS, Ryan DH, Boudreau MD, Windhauser MM, Tulley RT, Brooks ER, Bray GA. "Does vegetable oil attenuate the beneficial effects of fish oil in reducing risk factors for cardiovascular disease?" *Am J Clin Nutr.* 1997 Jul;66(1):89–96.

Ichikawa H, Aggarwal BB. "Guggulsterone inhibits osteoclastogenesis induced by receptor activator of nuclear factor-kappaB ligand and by tumor cells by suppressing nuclear factor-kappaB activation," *Clin Cancer Res.* 2006 Jan 15;12(2):662–68.

Ishiguro K, Ando T, Maeda O, Ohmiya N, Niwa Y, Kadomatsu K, Goto H. "Ginger ingredients reduce viability of gastric cancer cells via distinct mechanisms," *Biochem Biophys Res Commun.* 2007 Oct 12;362(1):218–23. Epub 2007 Aug 10.

Kakkar P, Singh BK. "Mitochondria: a hub of redox activities and cellular distress control," *Mol Cell Biochem.* 2007 Nov;305(1–2):235–53. Epub 2007 Jun 12.

Katiyar SK. "Green tea: a new option for the prevention or control of osteoarthritis," *Arthritis Res Ther.* 13.4(2011):121. Print.

Kris-Etherton PM, Grieger JA, Etherton TD. "Dietary reference intakes for DHA and EPA," *Prostaglandins Leukot Essent Fatty Acids.* 2009 Aug-Sep;81(2–3):99–104.

Kwon HM, Choi YJ, Choi JS, Kang SW, Bae JY, Kang IJ, Jun JG, Lee SS, Lim SS, Kang YH. "Blockade of cytokine-induced endothelial cell adhesion molecule expression by licorice isoliquiritigenin through NF-kappaB signal disruption," *Exp Biol Med (Maywood).* 2007 Feb;232(2):235–45.

Lee YR, Lee JH, Noh EM, Kim EK, Song MY, Jung WS, Park SJ, Kim JS, Park JW, Kwon KB, Park BH. "Guggulsterone blocks IL-1beta-mediated inflammatory responses by suppressing NF-kappaB activation in fibroblast-like synoviocytes," *Life Sci.* 2008 Jun 6:82 (23–24):1203–9.

Li B, Birdwell C. "Antithetic relationship of dietary arachidonic acid and eicosapentaenoic acid one icosanoid production in vivo," *J Lipid Res.* 1994 Oct;35(10):1869–77.

Li JJ, Gao RL. "Should atherosclerosis be considered a cancer of the vascular wall?" *Med Hypotheses.* 2005;64(4):694–98.

Li Q, Withoff S, Verma IM. "Inflammation-associated cancer: NF-kappaB is the lynchpin," *Trends Immunol.* 2005 Jun;26(6):318–25.

Li BY, Li XL, Gao HQ, Zhang JH, Cai Q, Cheng M, Lu M. "Grape seed procyanidin B2 inhibits advanced glycation end product-induced endothelial cell apoptosis through regulating GSK3β phosphorylation," *Cell Biol Int.* 2011 Jul;35(7):663–69.

Liu FC, Hung LF, Wu WL, Chang DM, Huang CY, Lai JH, Ho LJ. "Chondroprotective effects and mechanisms of resveratrol in advanced glycation end products-stimulated chondrocytes," *Arthritis Res Ther.* 2010;12(5):R167. Epub 2010 Sep 8.

Lopez-Armada MJ, Carames B, Martin MA, Cillero-Pastor B, Lires-Dean M, Fuentes-Boquete I, Arenas J, Bianco, FJ. "Mitochondrial activity is modulated by TNFalpha and IL-1beta in normal human chondrocyte cells," *Osteoarthritis Cartilage.* 2006 Oct;14(10):1011–22. Epub 2006 May 5.

Lv N. "Guggulsterone, a plant sterol, inhibits NFKB activation and protects pancreatic beta cells from cytokine toxicity," *Mol Cell Endocrinol.* 2008 July 16:289(1–2):49–59.

Malekinejad H, Rezabakhsh A, Rahmani F, Hobbenaghi R. "Silymarin regulates the cytochrome P450 3A2 and glutathione peroxides in the liver of streptozotocin-induced diabetic rats," *Phytomedicine.* 2012 May 15;19(7):583–90. Epub 2012 Mar 24.

Manna SK, Mukhopadhyay A, Aggarwal BB. "Resveratrol suppresses TNF-induced activation of nuclear transcription factors NF-kappa B, activator protein-1, and apoptosis: potential role of reactive oxygen intermediates and lipid peroxidation," *J Immunol.* 2000 Jun 15;164(12):6509–19.

McCann SM, Mastronardi C, de Laurentiis A, Rettori V. "The nitric oxide theory of aging revisited," *Ann N Y Acad Sci.* 2005 Dec;1057:64–84.

Milne JC, Lambert PD, Schenk S, Carney DP, Smith JJ, Gagne DJ, Jin L, Boss O, Perni RB, Vu CB, Bernis JE, Xie R, Disch JS, Ng PY, Nunes JJ, Lynch AV, Yang H, Galonek H, Israelian K, Choy W, Iffland A, Lavu S, Medvedik O, Sinclair DA, Olefsky JM, Jirousek MR, Elliott PJ, Westphal CH. "Small molecule activators of SIRT1 as therapeutics for the treatment of type 2 diabetes," *Nature.* 2007 Nov 29;450(7170):712–16.

Monfort J, Martel-Pelletier J, Pelletier JP. "Chondroitin sulphate for symptomatic osteoarthritis: critical appraisal of meta-analyses," *Curr Med Res Opin.* 2008 May;24(5):1303–8.

Moussaieff A, Shohami E, Kashman Y, Fride E, Schmitz ML, Renner F, Fiebich BL, Munoz E, Ben-Neriah Y, Mechoulam R. "Incensole acetate, a novel anti-inflammatory compound isolated from Boswellia resin, inhibits nuclear factor-kappa B activation," *Mol Pharmacol.* 2007 Dec;72(6):1657–64.

Neelands PJ, Clandinin MT. "Diet fat influences liver plasma membrane lipid composition and glucagon-stimulated adenylate cyclase activity," *Biochem J.* 1983;(212):573–83.

Orrenius S. "Reactive oxygen species in mitochondria-mediated cell death," *Drug Metab Rev.* 2007;39(2–3):443–55.

Orrenius S, Gogvadze V, Zhivotovsky B. "Mitochondrial oxidative stress: implications for cell death," *Ann Rev Pharmacol Toxicol.* 2007;47:143–83.

Ottestad I, Hassani S, Borge GI, Kohler A, Vogt G, Hyötyläinen T, Orešič M, Brønner KW, Holven KB, Ulven SM, Myhrstad MC. "Fish oil supplementation alters the plasma lipidomic profile and increases long-chain PUFAs of phospholipids and triglycerides in healthy subjects," *PLoS One.* 2012;7(8):e42550. Epub 2012 Aug 28.

Pae HO, Jeong SO, Kim HS, Kim SH, Song YS, Kim SK, Chai KY, Chung HT. "Dimethoxycurcumin, a synthetic curcumin analogue with higher metabolic stability, inhibits NO production, inducible NO synthase expression and NF-kappaB activation in RAW264.7 macrophages activated with LPS," *Mol Nutr Food Res.* 2008 Sep;52(9):1082–91.

Pavelka K, Gatterova J, Olejarova M, Machacek S, Giacovelli G, Rovati LC. "Glucosamine sulfate use and delay of progression of knee osteoarthritis: a 3-year randomized, placebo-controlled, double-blind study," *Arch Intern Med.* 2002 Oct 14;162(18):2113–23.

Rasheed Z, Anbazhagan AN, Akhtar N, Ramamurthy S, Voss FR, Haqqi TM. "Green tea polyphenol epigallocatechin-3-gallate inhibits advanced glycation end product-induced expression of tumor necrosis factor-alpha and matrix metalloproteinase-13 in human chondrocytes," *Arthritis Res Ther.* 2009;11(3):R71.

Richards JB, Valdes AM, Gardner JP, Paximadas D, Kimura M. "Higher serum vitamin D concentrations are associated with longer leukocyte telomere length in women," *Am J Clin Nutr.* 2007 Nov;86(5):1420-25.

Roskoski R Jr, Herbert JD. *Biochemistry review.* Saunders, 1996.

Roy S, Khanna S, Krishnaraju AV, Subbaraju GV, Yasmin T, Bagchi D, Sen CK. "Regulation of vascular responses to inflammation: inducible matrix metalloproteinase-3 expression in human microvascular endothelial cells is sensitive to antiinflammatory Boswellia," *Antioxid Redox Signal.* 2006 Mar-Apr;8(3-4):653-60.

Sarris J, Kavanagh DJ, Byrne G, Bone KM, Adams J, Deed G. "The Kava Anxiety Depression Spectrum Study (KADSS): a randomized, placebo-controlled crossover trial using an aqueous extract of Piper methysticum," *Psychopharmacology (Berl).* 2009 Aug;205(3):399-407. Epub 2009 May 9.

Sawitzke AD, Shi H, Finco MF, Dunlop DD, Harris CL, Singer NG, Bradley JD, Silver D, Jackson CG, Lane NE, Oddis CV, Wolfe F, Lisse J, Furst DE, Bingham CO, Reda DJ, Moskowitz RW, Williams HJ, Clegg DO. "Clinical efficacy and safety of glucosamine, chondroitin sulphate, their combination, celecoxib or placebo taken to treat osteoarthritis of the knee: 2-year results from GAIT," *Ann Rheum Dis.* 2010 Aug;69(8):1459-64. doi: 10.1136/ard.2009.120469. Epub 2010 Jun 4.

Scholtissen S, Bruyere O, Neuprez A, Severens JL, Herrero-Beaumont G, Rovati L, Hiligsmann M, Reginster JY. "Glucosamine sulphate in the treatment of knee osteoarthritis: cost-effectiveness comparison with paracetamol," *Int J Clin Pract.* 2010;64(6):756-62.

Serhan CN, Arita M, Hong S, Gotlinger K. "Resolvins, docosatrienes, and neuroprotectins, novel omega-3-derived mediators, and their endogenous aspirin-triggered epimers," *Lipids.* 2004;39(11):1125-32.

Shishodia S, Majumdar S, Banerjee S, Aggarwal BB. "Ursolic acid inhibits nuclear factor-kappaB activation induced by carcinogenic agents through suppression of IkappaBalpha kinase and p65 phosphorylation: correlation with down-regulation of cyclooxygenase 2, matrix metalloproteinase 9, and cyclin D1," *Cancer Res.* 2003 Aug 1;63(15):4375-83.

Shishodia S. "Guggulsterone inhibits NF-kappaB and IkappaBalpha kinase activation, suppresses expression of anti-apoptotic gene products, and enhances apoptosis," *J Biol Chem.* 2004 Nov 5;279(45):47148-58.

Siemoneit U, Hofmann B, Kather N, Lamkemeyer T, Madlung J, Franke L, Schneider G, Jauch J, Poeckel D, Werz O. "Identification and functional analysis of cyclooxygenase-1 as a molecular target of boswellic acids," *Biochem Pharmacol.* 2008 Jan 15;75(2):503-13. Epub 2007 Sep 14.

Takada Y, Bhardwaj A, Potdar P, Aggarwal BB. "Nonsteroidal anti-inflammatory agents differ in their ability to suppress NF-kappaB activation, inhibition of expression of cyclo-oxygenase-2 and cyclin D1, and abrogation of tumor cell proliferation," *Oncogene.* 2004 Dec 9;23(57):9247-58.

Terkeltaub R, Johnson K, Murphy A, Ghosh S. "Invited review: the mitochondrion in osteo-arthritis," *Mitochondrion.* 2002 Feb;1(4):301-19.

Teschke R, Genthner A, Wolff A. "Kava hepatotoxicity: comparison of aqueous, etha-nolic, acetonic kava extracts and kava-herbs mixtures," *J Ethnopharmacol.* 2009 Jun 25;123(3):378-84. Epub 2009 Apr 5.

Teschke R, Sarris J, Schweitzer I. "Kava hepatotoxicity in traditional and modern use: the presumed Pacific kava paradox hypothesis revisited," *Br J Clin Pharmacol.* 2012 Feb;73(2):170-74. doi: 10.1111/j.1365-2125.2011.04070.x.

Uebelhart D. "Clinical review of chondroitin sulfate in osteoarthritis," *Osteoarthritis Cartilage.* 2008;16 Suppl 3:S19-S21.

Vidgren HM, Agren JJ, Schwab U, Rissanen T, Hänninen O, Uusitupa MI. "Incorporation of n-3 fatty acids into plasma lipid fractions, and erythrocyte membranes and platelets during dietary supplementation with fish, fish oil, and docosahexaenoic acid-rich oil among healthy young men," *Lipids.* 1997 Jul;32(7):697-705.

Wilcox RB. *High Yield Biochemistry.* Lippincott Williams & Wilkins, 1999.

Yin MJ, Yamamoto Y, Gaynor RB. "The anti-inflammatory agents aspirin and salicylate inhibit the activity of I(kappa)B kinase-beta," *Nature.* 1998 Nov 5;396(6706):77-80.

Zadshir A, Tareen N, Pan D, Norris K, Martins D. "The prevalence of hypovitaminosis D among US adults; data from the NHANES III," *Ethn Dis.* 2005 Autumn;15(4 Suppl 5): S5-97-101.

APPENDIX II

How the *Healthy Joints for Life* Lifestyle Works To Battle Heart Disease and Decrease Cancer Risk

Arterburn LM, Hall EB, Oken H. "Distribution, interconversion, and dose response of n-3 fatty acids in humans," *Am J Clin Nutr.* 2006 Jun;83(6 Suppl):1467S-1476S.

Bernstein L, Henderson BE, Hanisch R, Sullivan-Halley J, Ross RK. "Physical exer-cise and reduced risk of breast cancer in young women," *J Natl Cancer Inst.* 1994 Sep 21;86(18):1403-8.

Bingham SA, Pignatelli B, Pollock JR, Ellul A, Malaveille C, Gross G, Runswick S, Cummings JH, O'Neill IK. "Does increased endogenous formation of N-nitroso compounds in the human colon explain the association between red meat and colon cancer?" *Carcinogenesis.* 1996 Mar;17(3):515-23.

Brace LD. "Cardiovascular benefits of garlic (Allium sativum L)," *J Cardiovasc Nurs.* 2002 Jul;16(4):33-49.

Daley CA, Abbott A, Doyle PS, Nader GA, Larson S. "A review of fatty acid profiles and antioxidant content in grass-fed and grain-fed beef," *Nutr Journ.* 2010;9:10.

Ding EL, Hutfless SM, Ding X, Girotra S. "Chocolate and prevention of cardiovascular disease: a systematic review," *Nutr Metab (Lond).* 2006 Jan 3;3:2.

Duncker DJ, Bache RJ. "Regulation of coronary blood flow during exercise," *Physiol Rev.* 2008 Jul;88(3):1009-86.

Hunter JE, Zhang J, Kris-Etherton PM. "Cardiovascular disease risk of dietary stearic acid compared with trans, other saturated, and unsaturated fatty acids: a systematic review," *Am J Clin Nutr.* 2010 Jan;91(1):46-63.

Hsieh TC, Wu JM. "Resveratrol: Biological and pharmaceutical properties as anticancer molecule," *Biofactors.* 2010 Sep-Oct;36(5):360-9.

Kenfield S, Meir J, Stampfer M, Giovannucci E, Chan J. "Physical activity and survival after prostate cancer diagnosis in the health professionals follow-up study," *J Clin Oncol.* 2011 Feb 20;29(6):726-32.

Kwon GT, Cho HJ, Chung WY, Park KK, Moon A, Park JH. "Isoliquiritigenin inhibits migration and invasion of prostate cancer cells: possible mediation by decreased JNK/AP-1 signaling," *J Nutr Biochem.* 2009 Sep;20(9):663-76.

Leung FP, Yung LM, Laher I, Yao X, Chen ZY, Huant Y. "Exercise, vascular wall and cardiovascular diseases: an update (Part 1)," *Sports Med.* 2008;28(12):1009-24.

Mozaffarian D, Rimm EB, Herrington DM. "Dietary fats, carbohydrate, and progression of coronary atherosclerosis in postmenopausal women," *Am J Clin Nutr.* 2004 Nov;80(5):1175-84.

Mozaffarian D, Katan MB, Ascherio A, Stampfer MJ, Willett WC. "Trans fatty acids and cardiovascular disease," *N Engl J Med.* 2006 Apr 13;354(15):1601-13.

Myers J. "Exercise and Cardiovascular Health," *Circulation.* 2003;107:e2.

Myers J, Prakash M, Froelicher V, et al. "Exercise capacity and mortality among men referred for exercise testing," *N Engl J Med.* 2002;346:793-801.

Norat T, et al. "Meat, fish, and colorectal cancer risk: the european prospective investigation into cancer and nutrition," *J Natl Cancer Inst.* (15 June 2005);97(12):906-16.

Saha A, Kuzuhara T, Echigo N, Suganuma M, Fujiki H. "New role of (-)-epicatechin in enhancing the induction of growth inhibition and apoptosis in human lung cancer cells by curcumin," *Cancer Prev Res* (Phila Pa). 2010 Aug;3(8):953-62.

Sonestedt E, Ericson U, Gullberg B, Skog K, Olsson H, Wirfält E. "Do both heterocyclic amines and omega-6 polyunsaturated fatty acids contribute to the incidence of breast cancer in postmenopausal women of the Malmö diet and cancer cohort?" *The International Journal of Cancer.* (UICC International Union Against Cancer) 2008;123(7):1637-43.

Stampfer MF, Hu FB, Manson JE, Rimm EB, Willett WC. "Primary prevention of coronary heart disease in women through diet and lifestyle," *N Engl J Med.* 2000 Jul 6;343(1):16-22.

Vidgren HM, Agren JJ, Schwab U, Rissanen T, Hänninen O, Uusitupa MI. "Incorporation of n-3 fatty acids into plasma lipid fractions, and erythrocyte membranes and platelets during dietary supplementation with fish, fish oil, and docosahexaenoic acid-rich oil among healthy young men," *Lipids*. 1997 Jul;32(7):697-705.

Virtanen JK, Mozaffarian D, Chiuve SE, Rimm EB. "Fish consumption and risk of major chronic disease in men," *Am J Clin Nutr*. 2008 Dec;88(6):1618-25.

Wang YT, Wang J, Zhao M, DI HJ. "Inhibitory effects of reduced glutathione sodium on renal nuclear factor-kappaB expression in rats with diabetes of different stages," *Nan Fang Yi Ke Da Xue Xue Bao*. 2007 Mar;27(3):332-35.

Wang P, Aronson WJ, Huang M, Zhang Y, Lee RP, Heber D, Henning SM. "Green tea polyphenols and metabolites in prostatectomy tissue: implications for cancer prevention," *Cancer Prev Res (Phila Pa)*. 2010 Aug;3(8):985-93.

Wolin KY, Yan Y, Colditz GA, Lee I-M. "Physical activity and colon cancer prevention: a meta-analysis," *Br J Cancer*. 2009;100:611-16.

Wyshak G, Frisch RE. "Breast cancer among former college athletes compared to non-athletes: a 15-year follow-up," *Br J Cancer*. 2000 Feb;82(3):726-30.

Yung LM, Laher I, Yao X, Chen ZY, Huang Y, Leung FP. "Exercise, vascular wall and cardiovascular diseases: an update (part 2)," *Sports Med*. 2009;39(1):45-63.

Zahid M, Saeed M, Ali MF, Rogan EG, Cavalieri EL. "N-acetylcysteine blocks formation of cancer-initiating estrogen-DNA adducts in cells," *Free Radic Biol Med*. 2010 Aug 1;49(3):392-400.

INDEX

ACKNOWLEDGMENTS

I'D LIKE TO ACKNOWLEDGE THE EFFORTS OF THE MANY PEOPLE who played an important role in this project. This was a labor of love. And without strong motivation it never would have materialized.

I'd first like to thank my late mother, who struggled with her battle with arthritis; my patients, who count on me to do what is best for them; and my former teammates, who live with the battle scars of the great game of football, for providing me with the motivation to spend countless hours researching, writing, and rewriting.

I'd like to thank all my coaches in both football and baseball, who ingrained the value of hard work into my fabric. I am a product of their teachings. I'd especially like to thank Coach Carm Cozza for the permission to use some of the stories he has told so well about the people and days when I played football at Yale.

I'd like to thank Gerry Combs for her diligent typing of the first draft and the bibliography, which was so technical, it probably made her hair curl. I'd also like to thank my nurse and secretary, Cathy Dudeff, for all of her assistance throughout this project. My life would not be nearly as efficient or enjoyable without her.

Thanks to my lifelong friend John Bonadies, M.D., who reviewed the entire initial manuscript and gave me countless suggestions, all in red Magic Marker. Without his initial encouragement this book would not have come to fruition.

To my best friend at Yale, Ron Darling, who took freshman English with me and years later read my initial manuscript without reminding me that he earned an A and I didn't.

Thank you to my friend and lawyer Edward Walsh, who helped me with contracts and talked sense into me on numerous occasions.

Special gratitude must be extended to Nick Perricone, M.D., who, as a noted bestselling medical author, met with me and coached me through the process and science.

Deep thanks to my good friend interventional cardiologist and author Stephen Sinatra, M.D., and his wonderful wife, Jan Sinatra, R.N., who provided me with encouragement and reviewed draft number two, putting forth far-reaching suggestions. They lent their time liberally and without expectations. Their mark is most certainly on this book.

Thanks to Kit Kiefer, who explained to me that draft two was an important book written completely wrong. He helped contour the book so that the public could read it, and was an absolute pleasure to work with.

Thank you to my friend John Raybin for introducing me to Kit and to Arthur and Elaine Haut, who helped convince my literary agent, Faith Hamlin, that this project was worthwhile.

Thank you to my literary agent, Faith Hamlin, for taking a chance on a first-time author who didn't seem to meet any of the criteria to merit her representation. She treated me gently yet sternly, guiding me in the right direction on every front. I look forward to a long and fruitful relationship.

My extreme gratitude goes out to my coauthor, Sheila Curry Oakes, for spending countless hours further reformatting and reorganizing the entire book into a coherent and cohesive prescriptive program. She patiently forced me to clarify, substantiate, and simplify. Ever so quietly, she made the book better and did so without injuring my psyche. I greatly admire her tact, reason, and creative writing skills.

Thanks to art professor Pete Bonadies for introducing me to my fantastic illustrator, Janet Croog. His suggestions and keen eye are deeply appreciated.

Thanks to Janet Croog, who turned my ideas into the wonderful characters in the exercises in Chapter 5. She is an amazing young artist with a unique combination of creativity, affability, and diligence.

To Deb Brody, Rebecca Hunt and the talented people at Harlequin, who saw potential in this project and supported it enthusiastically. Being an orthopedic surgeon and writing a book on the nonsurgical treatment of joint pain seemed contradictory to many publishers. Deb Brody saw the concept in a completely different manner, understanding that any surgeon recommending a nonsurgical treatment must be absolutely convinced of its veracity. What seemed to be a deterrent to some became a selling point to Deb and Harlequin. They understood that the best surgeons do surgery very well, but in fact do their best to help patients avoid surgery.

And thanks to my family for allowing this project, at times, to dominate our lives. My wife, son, and daughter all sacrificed for this book. My absence was conspicuous to each of them. And I know that wasn't fair. All three were patient, especially when "Daddy was grumpy writing his book." Each of them listened or read portions of the book and supplied important feedback. My wife was particularly understanding of my mission, those late nights, early mornings, and missed "dates." I couldn't have written this book and my life wouldn't be as fulfilling without them.

ABOUT THE AUTHOR

RICHARD DIANA, M.D., IS A HIGHLY TRAINED ORTHOPEDIC surgeon specializing in arthroscopic knee and shoulder surgery. His specialized surgical training, when combined with his history as an NFL football player and a collegiate football and baseball All-American, uniquely positions him among his peers.

Dr. Diana also has a keen interest in the nonsurgical treatment of joint pain. He strongly believes in integrating mainstream medical techniques with the use of less conventional treatments, including diet regulation, exercise, and supplements. His structured protocols have been honed over a twenty-year career as a practicing orthopedic surgeon and are supported by scientific evidence.

He graduated cum laude from Yale University in 1982 with a degree in molecular biophysics and biochemistry. It is upon this foundation that his interest in the molecular nature of joint pain rests. Upon graduation he was one of Yale's most celebrated student athletes, receiving numerous Yale and national distinctions, including CoSIDA, the Hartford and Miller Lite Beer Consensus Football All-American honors. He was a GTE Football Academic All-American and one of twelve scholar athletes recognized by The National Football Foundation and College Football Hall of Fame. In baseball he was selected as an honorable mention All-American, as well as All Ivy and All Eastern Intercollegiate Baseball League. No other orthopedic surgeon has been named both first team Division I Football All-American and Academic All-American.

After graduation he was drafted by the Miami Dolphins and

played in Super Bowl XVII. He retired from the NFL to attend the Yale School of Medicine, from which he graduated in 1987. He completed his orthopedic residency training at Yale–New Haven Hospital and then received fellowship certification in orthopedic sports medicine at the University of Massachusetts Medical Center from longtime Boston Red Sox team physician Arthur Pappas, M.D. After completing his fellowship, he worked with the Boston Red Sox for six years as an orthopedic consultant.

Dr. Diana is board certified by the American Board of Orthopaedic Surgery and is a member of the American Academy of Orthopaedic Surgeons. In 2006 and in each consecutive year he was named to Dr. Stephen Sinatra's esteemed Top 100 Doctors in America. He has been in practice with Connecticut Orthopaedic Specialists (www.ct-ortho.com) since 1993 and has been one of the managing partners since 1995. Dr. Diana is currently a clinical instructor at the Yale School of Medicine, and an attending surgeon at Yale–New Haven Hospital. He is, or has been, a collegiate orthopedic sports consultant at Yale University, Quinnipiac University, and Southern Connecticut State University and a high school orthopedic sports consultant at many local high schools. He has been published in the medical literature.

Through generous volunteer work, charitable gifts, and the Diana Family Charitable Trust, Dr. Diana continues to play an active and enthusiastic role in the community. Dr. Diana lives in Hamden, Connecticut, with his wife and children.

Through his book *Healthy Joints for Life* Dr. Diana hopes to be able to extend his unique expertise on the nonconventional treatment of joint pain to a large population, one that he otherwise would not be able to reach.

Visit his websites: www.richdianamd.com and www.healthyjointsforlife.com.